Dentistry and Oral Sciences

nova
Medicine & Health
New York

Dentistry and Oral Sciences

Multiple Choice Questions on Oral Medicine and Radiology – A Rapid Review in Dentistry
Karthik Rajaram Mohan
Ravikumar Pethagounder Thangavel
Saramma Mathew Fenn
2022. ISBN: 978-1-68507-584-2

A Compendium of Principles and Practices of Laser Biophotonics in Oral Medicine
Fakir Mohan Debta (Editor)
Ekagrata Mishraa (Editor)
Neha Patyal (Editor)
2022. ISBN: 978-1-68507-441-8 (Hardcover)

Laser Light Therapy in Dentistry: Efficacy, Uses and Limitations
Georgios E. Romanos, DDS, PhD (Editor)
2022. ISBN: 978-1-68507-068-7 (Hardcover)
2022. ISBN: 978-1-68507-345-9 (eBook)

Platelet Concentrates in Periodontal Therapy: An Update
Diksha Ramesh Agrawal (Editor)
Priyanka Ganesh Jaiswal, PhD (Editor)
2021. ISBN: 978-1-53619-688-7 (eBook)

Dentistry: Advances in Research and Future Directions
Kirti Chawla (Editor)
Lata Goyal (Editor)
2021. ISBN: 978-1-53619-042-7 (Hardcover)
2021. ISBN: 978-1-53619-088-5 (eBook)

Critical Thoughts on Oral Lichen Planus
Dante Antonio Migliari, DDS, PhD (Editor)
Silvio Kenji Hirota, DDS, PhD (Editor)
2021. ISBN: 978-1-53618-897-4 (eBook)

More information about this series can be found at https://novapublishers.com/product-category/series/microbiology-research-advances/

Karthik Rajaram Mohan,
Ravikumar Pethagounder Thangavel
and Saramma Mathew Fenn

Multiple Choice Questions in Oral Medicine and Radiology

A Rapid Review in Dentistry

nova
Medicine & Health
New York

DOI: https://doi.org/10.52305/AZYT1272

Library of Congress Cataloging-in-Publication Data

ISBN: 978-1-68507-584-2

Published by Nova Science Publishers, Inc. † New York

Contents

Preface

This book contains a series of multiple choice questions on oral medicine and radiology that will be helpful for undergraduates and postgraduates in the field of dentistry, as well as undergraduates who are applying for licensure examinations like NEET, USMLE, and National Board examinations.

Acknowledgments

I sincerely owe my gratitude to the Almighty and the constant support by my father Dr. Rajaram Mohan MD, DPM (Psy), mother Kasthuri, sister Kavitha, brother R. Rajkumar, spouse M/s Dr. J. Aruna devi. B.D.S and my daughter K. Diya and my aspiring teacher Capt. Dr. Elangovan Somasundaram. MDS and all other faculties of Vinayaka mission's Sankarachariyar Dental College, Salem in enduring constant support for the outcome of this book, which helps undergraduate and postgraduate students in dentistry.

Part 1. Oral Medicine

Chapter 1

Terminologies in Oral Medicine

Questions

1. An abnormal mass of tissue, the growth of which exceeds that of the adjacent tissue and persists in the same excessive manner even after the cessation of stimuli, which evoked the change is called?
   a. Swelling
   b. Cyst
   c. Neoplasm
   d. Abscess

2. A pathological cavity lined by epithelium and is covered by fluid, semifluid or gaseous material is called?
   a. Swelling
   b. Neoplasm
   c. Abscess
   d. Cyst

3. The flat and well-circumscribed lesions that are noticeable because of their colour change from usual are called?
   a. Papule
   b. Macule
   c. Plaques
   d. Pustules

4. The raised solid lesions greater than 1cm in diameter are called?
   a. Plaques
   b. Papule
   c. Macule
   d. Nodule

5. Raised solid lesions smaller than 1cm in diameter are called?
   a. Papule
   b. Plaque
   c. Macule
   d. Nodule

6. Fluid-filled elevated lesions less than 1cm in diameter are called?
   a. Bulla
   b. Vesicle
   c. Nodule
   d. Plaque

7. Fluid-filled elevated lesions greater than 1cm in diameter are called?
   a. Bulla
   b. Vesicle
   c. Nodule
   d. Plaque

8. The red lesions often caused by the rupture of vesicles or bullae, usually by trauma, are called?
   a. Nodule
   b. Papule
   c. Erosion
   d. Blister

9. What is the pin-point haemorrhages less than 0.5 cm caused by leakage of blood into the connective tissue is called?
   a. Petechiae
   b. Papule
   c. Hematoma
   d. Ecchymosis

10. The break-in continuity of epithelium brought about by molecular destruction and is covered by a granulation tissue is called?
   a. Ulcer
   b. Ecchymosis
   c. Petechiae
   d. Blister

11. The abnormal collection of blood outside the blood vessel?
   a. Papilloma
   b. Fibroma
   c. Hematoma
   d. Petechiae

12. The flat discoloured area caused by leakage of blood from damaged capillaries into the surrounding tissue is called?
   a. Ecchymoses
   b. Hematoma
   c. Petechiae
   d. Papilloma

13. The asymptomatic, 1-3mm well-circumscribed, tan or brown coloured macule often seen on sun-exposed areas of skin are called?
    a. Freckle
    b. Epulis
    c. Granuloma
    d. Papule

14. The growth resulting from a proliferation of blood vessels is?
    a. Angioma
    b. Papilloma
    c. Granuloma
    d. Teratoma

15. The gland-like cells of the epithelial tissue that covers organs, glands, and other structures within the body are called?
    a. Angioma
    b. Papilloma
    c. Adenoma
    d. Teratoma

16. A benign epithelial tumour that grows exophytic with finger-like projections on its surface?
    a. Adenoma
    b. Papilloma
    c. Teratoma
    d. Angioma

17. Tumours composed of tissues that are generally not present at the site?
    a. Teratoma
    b. Angioma
    c. Adenoma
    d. Papilloma

18. A tumour like malformation containing tissues naïve to the site is called?
    a. Hamartoma
    b. Angioma
    c. Papilloma
    d. Adenoma

19. The tumour that can arise from fibrous connective tissue and grow in all organs?
    a. Fibroma
    b. Lipoma
    c. Adenoma
    d. Papilloma

20. A benign tumour made up of fat or adipose tissue?
    a. Fibroma
    b. Lipoma
    c. Adenoma
    d. Papilloma

21. A tumour that is produced from pigment-producing melanocytes?
    a. Fibroma
    b. Lipoma
    c. Melanoma
    d. Angioma

22. A tumour of bone marrow, where there is a clonal proliferation of plasma cells causing abnormal proteins in urine and blood?
    a. Fibroma
    b. Lipoma
    c. Teratoma
    d. Myeloma

23. A malignant tumour of connective tissue such as muscle, joint?
    a. Sarcoma
    b. Melanoma
    c. Teratoma
    d. Lipoma

24. A tumour formed on a nerve cell sheath?
    a. Sarcoma
    b. Neuroma
    c. Lipoma
    d. Melanoma

25. Tumour is made up of cartilage and forms in bone or soft tissue?
    a. Chondroma
    b. Neuroma
    c. Myeloma
    d. Fibroma

26. A benign tumour arising from smooth muscle such as the uterus or gastrointestinal tract?
    a. Leiomyoma
    b. Chondroma
    c. Neuroma
    d. Myxoma

27. A tumour consisting of myxomatous connective tissue mucin containing acid mucopolysaccharides like hyaluronic acid and chondroitin sulphate?
    a. Neuroma
    b. Angioma
    c. Myxoma
    d. Melanoma

28. A Vascular tumour composed of spindle cells derived from Pericytes?
    a. Neuroma
    b. Perithelioma
    c. Myxoma
    d. Melanoma

29. The mass of clotted blood forms in tissue, organs or body spaces due to damaged blood vessels?
    a. Haematoma
    b. Teratoma
    c. Myxoma
    d. Myeloma

30. A benign mesenchymal tumour of striated muscle origin?
    a. Rhabdomyoma
    b. Leiomyoma
    c. Myeloma
    d. Melanoma

Answers

1. c. Neoplasm.
2. d. Cyst.
3. b. Macule.
4. a. Plaques.
5. a. Papule.
6. b. Vesicle.
7. a. Bulla.
8. c. Erosion.
9. a. Petechiae.
10. a. Ulcer.
11. c. Haematoma.
12. a. Ecchymoses.
13. a. Freckle.
14. a. Angioma.
15. c. Adenoma.
16. b. Papilloma.
17. a. Teratoma.
18. a. Hamartoma.
19. a. Fibroma.
20. b. Lipoma.
21. c. Melanoma.
22. d. Myeloma.
23. a. Sarcoma.
24. b. Neuroma.
25. a. Chondroma.
26. a. Leiomyoma.
27. c. Myxoma.
28. b. Perithelioma.
29. a. Haematoma.
30. a. Rhabdomyoma.

Chapter 2

White Lesions of the Oral Cavity

Questions

1. The following are the reasons for white lesions in the oral cavity, except?
   a. Increased production of keratin
   b. Imbibition of water molecules by oral epithelium
   c. Oral mucosa exposed to Toxic chemicals
   d. Thinning of stratum spinosum

2. Does the Pseudo membrane comprise the following?
   a. Fungal Mycelium, Neutrophils, Sloughed epithelial cells
   b. Fungal Mycelium, Neutrophils, epithelial cells
   c. Fungal Mycelium, Basophils, Sloughed Epithelial cells
   d. Fungal Mycelium, Basophils, Epithelial cells

3. The predisposing factors for oral candidiasis include the intake of all the following drugs except?
   a. Immunosuppressive drugs
   b. Chemotherapeutic drugs
   c. Antibiotic drugs
   d. Haematinics

4. The local predisposing factors for oral candidiasis include all the following except.
   a. Smoking
   b. Chronic denture wearing
   c. Hypersalivation
   d. Topical steroids

5. The penetration of candida yeast into the epithelial cells is facilitated with the help of the following?
   a. Ligases
   b. Lipases
   c. Mitochondria
   d. Cytoplasm

6. The following are the associated candida lesions except?
   a. Denture stomatitis
   b. Angular cheilitis
   c. Median Rhomboid Glossitis
   d. Lichen planus

7. The most common area affected by Erythematous candidiasis is?
   a. Alveolar mucosa
   b. Gingiva
   c. Hard palate
   d. Vermilion border of lip

8. The most common type of candidiasis encountered in HIV patients is all, except?
   a. Erythematous candidiasis
   b. Pseudomembranous candidiasis
   c. Chronic hyperplastic candidiasis
   d. Nodular candidiasis

9. The malignant transformation associated with chronic plaque-type and nodular candidiasis is hypothesised due to the capacity of candida yeasts to produce?
   a. Nitrosamine
   b. Carbon
   c. Polycyclic aromatic hydrocarbon
   d. Chondroitin sulphate

10. Does chronic mucocutaneous candidiasis occur in the following endocrine abnormalities?
    a. Hyperparathyroidism and Addison's disease
    b. Hypoparathyroidism and Cushing's disease
    c. Hypothyroidism and Addisons disease
    d. Hyperthyroidism and Cushing's disease

11. Which white lesion is used as a marker of HIV disease activity since it is associated with low CD4+ cell counts?
    a. Hairy Leukoplakia
    b. Nodular Leukoplakia
    c. Speckled Leukoplakia
    d. Non homogeneous Leukoplakia

12. The following white lesion that has a cracked mud-like appearance is?
    a. Nodular Leukoplakia
    b. Homogeneous Leukoplakia
    c. Non-Homogeneous Leukoplakia
    d. Candidal Leukoplakia

13. The type of leukoplakia in which numerous papillary projections are seen?
    a. Homogeneous Leukoplakia
    b. Non-Homogeneous Leukoplakia
    c. Proliferative Verrucous Leukoplakia
    d. Speckled Leukoplakia

14. A chronic, insidious disease affecting any part of the oral cavity, including the pharynx and upper one-third of the oesophagus, characterised by progressive fibrosis and gradual inability to open the mouth?
    a. Leukoplakia
    b. Candidiasis
    c. Oral submucous fibrosis
    d. Lichen planus

15. The primary etiological factor for oral submucous fibrosis is?
    a. Arecoline
    b. Xylocaine
    c. Xylitol
    d. Carboxymethyl cellulose

16. The characteristic appearance of oral mucosa affected by oral submucous fibrosis is described as the following?
    a. Ebbing tide appearance
    b. Cracked mud appearance
    c. Fruit-laden appearance
    d. Marbling appearance

17. Does the white lesion represent a delayed hypersensitivity reaction to constituents derived from cinnamon flavoured denitrifies?
    a. Oral Lichenoid reactions
    b. Oral Lichen planus
    c. Oral Hairy Leukoplakia
    d. Oral submucous fibrosis

18. The following cells are mainly concerned with the development of oral lichen planus are?
    a. Autoreactive T lymphocytes
    b. Autoreactive B lymphocytes
    c. Reactive Eosinophils
    d. Reactive Basophils

19. The form of Lichen planus is characterised by the clinical appearance of a white circular-ring like pattern on the affected oral mucosa?
    a. Reticular Lichen planus
    b. Plaque like Lichen planus
    c. Annular Lichen planus
    d. Erosive lichen planus

20. The form of lichen planus is characterised by small white dots?
    a. Papular Lichen planus
    b. Annular Lichen planus.
    c. Erosive Lichen planus.
    d. Reticular Lichen planus.

21. The pruritic papules on the flexor surfaces of the arms and legs can provide relief by intense scratching that may aggravate the following sign or phenomenon referring to the lesions?
    a. Koebner Phenomenon.
    b. Nikolskys sign.
    c. Trousseau's sign.
    d. Auspitz's sign.

22. The etiopathogenesis of Graft vs Host Lichenoid reactions is mainly attributed to the interaction of stromal cells?
    a. Autoreactive T-Lymphocytes and Antigen Presenting cells (APC)
    b. Autoreactive B lymphocytes and Antigen Presenting cells (APC)
    c. Nonreactive T Lymphocytes and Antigen Presenting cells (APC)
    d. Nonreactive B lymphocytes and Antigen Presenting cells (APC)

23. Chronic Graft versus Host Disease is defined as the occurrence of more than the following day's post-Haematopoietic Stem cell Transplantation?
    a. 50 days
    b. 100 days
    c. 150 days
    d. 200 days

24. The autoantibodies present in Systemic Lupus Erythematosus involved the following except?
    a. Anti-neutrophil antibodies
    b. Anti-smith antibodies
    c. Anti-DNA antibodies
    d. SSA-Ro antibodies

25. The oral lesions of Discoid Lupus Erythematosus clinically differ from Systemic Lupus erythematosus in that?
    a. The white striae abruptly terminate in the centre with an erythematous area
    b. The white striae do not abruptly terminate in the centre with an erythematous area
    c. The central area of white striations ends abruptly in Peripheral white striations
    d. The central area of white striations does not end abruptly in Peripheral white striations

26. The subepithelial inflammation of T lymphocytes and neutrophilic granulocytes are part of abscess formed near the surface in patients with Psoriasis are termed?
    a. Phoenix abscess
    b. Cold abscess
    c. Munros microabscess
    d. Collar stud abscess

27. The characteristic veil-like white alteration of the mucosa disappears on stretching and reappears when the stretched mucosa is relieved?
    a. Leukedema
    b. Leukoplakia
    c. Lichen Planus
    d. Lupus Erythematosus

28. The chief alkaloid in Betel nut that causes fibrosis of the connective tissue of the oral cavity in oral submucous fibrosis is?
    a. Arecoline
    b. Acetylcholine
    c. Choline salicylate
    d. Slaked lime

29. Hyperacusis in advanced cases of oral submucous fibrosis is due to fibrosis of the following involvement of muscle?
    a. Stapedius
    b. Stylopharyngeus
    c. Hyoglossus
    d. Genioglossus

30. The Physiotherapy appliance with vernier calliper like measurement used in oral submucous fibrosis patients is?
    a. Therabyte Appliance
    b. Hawley Appliance
    c. Coffin's expander
    d. Hyrax Appliance

31. The surgical excision of fibrotic band in oral submucous fibrosis in advanced cases best excised by the following?
    a. Scalpel
    b. Diathermy
    c. Laser
    d. Bard parker blade.

32. The Breaking factor used in oral submucous fibrosis intralesional is?
    a. Collagenase.
    b. Hyaluronidase.
    c. Lipase.
    d. Maltase.

Answers

1. d. Thinning of stratum spinosum.
2. a. Fungal Mycelium, Neutrophils, sloughed epithelial cells.
3. d. Haematinics.
4. c. Hypersalivation.
5. b. Lipases.
6. d. Lichen Planus.
7. c. Hard Palate.
8. d. Nodular candidiasis.
9. a. Nitrosamine.
10. a. Hyperparathyroidism and Addison's Disease.
11. a. Hairy Leukoplakia.
12. b. Homogeneous Leukoplakia.
13. c. Proliferative Verrucous Leukoplakia.
14. c. Oral Submucous Fibrosis.
15. a. Arecoline.
16. d. Marbling Appearance.
17. a. Oral Lichenoid reactions.
18. a. Autoreactive T- Lymphocytes.
19. c. Annular Lichenplanus.
20. a. Papular Lichen Planus.
21. a. Koebner Phenomenon.
22. a. Autoreactive T-Lymphocytes and Antigen Presenting cells (APC).
23. b. 100 days.
24. d. SSA-Ro Antibodies.
25. a.The white striae abruptly terminate in the centre with the erythematous area.
26. c. Munro's Microabscess.
27. a. Leukoedema.
28. a. Arecoline.
29. a. Stapedius.
30. a. Therabyte appliance.
31. c. Laser.
32. b. Hyaluronidase.

Chapter 3

Red Lesions of the Oral Cavity

Questions

1. The following lesion appears red and has a velvety texture with a sharply defined margin?
   a. Leukoplakia
   b. Erythroplakia
   c. Oral submucous fibrosis
   d. Hyperplastic candidiasis

2. The red lesion formed by accidental ingestion of hot pizza?
   a. Pizza burn
   b. Chemical burn
   c. Hypochlorite accident
   d. Phenolic burn

3. The red lesion that occurs on the gingiva caused by allergy?
   a. Acute Gingivitis
   b. Chronic Gingivitis
   c. Plasma cell Gingivitis
   d. Scorbutic Gingivitis

4. The red lesion caused by chronic wearing of dentures and not removing them during night sleep?
   a. Denture stomatitis
   b. Chronic Hyperplastic candidiasis
   c. Acute Pseudomembranous candidiasis
   d. Nodular candidiasis.

5. The term "Erythroplakia of Queyrat" is derived from red lesions resembling cancer occurring in the following part?
   a. Penile skin
   b. Chest
   c. Neck
   d. Head

6. The red lesions caused by dilatation of capillaries often seen in the following systemic disorder?
   a. hereditary hemorrhagic telangiectasia
   b. Varix
   c. Ariboflavinosis
   d. Crohn's disease

7. The reddish nodular lesions on the hard palate in HIV patients?
   a. Kaposi sarcoma
   b. Wegener's Granulomatosis
   c. Purpura
   d. Petechiae.

8. The reddish depapillated areas due to change in size and shape and occur on the dorsum of the tongue?
   a. Erythema migrans
   b. Purpura
   c. Petechiae
   d. Kaposi sarcoma

9. The red lesion caused by diffuse bruising at the site of trauma?
   a. ecchymoses
   b. petechiae
   c. Purpura
   d. Varix

10. The small dilated veins on the ventral surface of the tongue seen among old or hypertensive patients?
   a. Lingual Varix
   b. Purpura
   c. Petechiae
   d. Ecchymoses

Answers

1. b. Erythroplakia.
2. a. Pizza burn.
3. c. Plasma cell Gingivitis.
4. a. Denture stomatitis.
5. a. Penile skin.
6. a. hereditary hemorrhagic telangiectasia.
7. a. Kaposi's sarcoma.
8. a. Erythema migrans.
9. a. Ecchymoses.
10. a. Lingual varix.

Chapter 4

Pigmented Lesions of the Oral Cavity

Questions

1. Melanin, the universal physiological pigment, is derived from the following amino acid?
   a. Valine.
   b. Leucine.
   c. Methionine.
   d. Tyrosine.

2. Which of the following arise because of melanocytic proliferation?
   a. Nevi.
   b. Freckle.
   c. Melanotic macule.
   d. Ephelis.

3. The dome-shaped appearance of naevus cells near the mucosal-submucosal junction is called?
   a. Compound nevi.
   b. Intramucosal nevi.
   c. Blue nevi.
   d. Naevi.

4. Which of the naevi are not derived from basal layer melanocytes?
   a. Blue naevi.
   b. Intramucosal naevi.
   c. Compound naevi.
   d. Junctional naevi.

5. The ABCDE criteria for clinical characteristics of Cutaneous Melanoma involves the following, EXCEPT?
   a. Asymmetry.
   b. Borders regular.
   c. Colour variegation.
   d. The diameter is greater than 6mm.

6. The following person gave the level of tumour involvement in the dermis for cutaneous Melanoma?
   a. Clarks.
   b. Fitzgerald.
   c. Black.
   d. Roentgen.

7. The following person gave the tumour thickness of Cutaneous Melanoma?
   a. Breslow.
   b. Clark.
   c. Fitzgerald.
   d. Roentgen.

8. The only clinicopathological subtype of Melanoma with a vertical growth phase?
   a. Superficial spreading.
   b. Lentigo malignant melanoma.
   c. Acral Lentiginous.
   d. Nodular Melanoma.

9. The ocular, dermal melanosis that usually involves the ophthalmic and Maxillary division of the Trigeminal nerve, with an increased risk of Glaucoma and uveal Melanoma, is called?
   a. Nevus of Ota.
   b. Nevus of Ito.
   c. Suns Nevus.
   d. Blue nevus.

10. The following nevus differs from nevus of Ota in that the pigmentation is distributed along the branches of Brachial nerves of the shoulder and posterior supraclavicular nerves?
    a. Nevus of Ito.
    b. blue nevus.
    c. Junctional nevus.
    d. Suns Nevus.

11. The treatment of choice for Nevus of Ota is?
    a. Pulsed Q-Switched Alexandrite Laser. (755 nm, 100ns).
    b. Diode Laser.
    c. Nd: Yag Laser.
    d. Co2 Laser.

12. The following term is known as the yellowish discolouration of the sclera?
    a. Carotenemia.
    b. Café-au-lait spots.
    c. Icterus.
    d. Launier Hunziker Pigmentation.

13. Café-au-lait spots (Coffee in cream or Coffee in Milk) Pigmentations are seen in the following disease?
    a. Von Recklinghausen's Disease.
    b. Mc Cune Albright's syndrome.
    c. Down syndrome.
    d. Melkerson Rosenthal syndrome.

14. The area of greyish pigmentation on the mucosa near silver amalgam restoration is called?
    a. Argyria.
    b. Burtonian line.
    c. Amalgam Tatoo.
    d. Carotenemia.

15. The term "Swift disease" refers to the pain and irritability of toes in infants, hypersalivation, the scarlet colouration of the cheek, nose due to the following element?
    a. Mercury.
    b. Silver.
    c. Lead.
    d. Gold.

16. The term that refers to facial pigmentation associated with pregnancy and using oral contraceptives is?
    a. Chloasma.
    b. blue nevus.
    c. Sun nevus.
    d. Graphite tattoo.

17. A common acquired autoimmune disorder associated with hypomelanosis is?
    a. Vitiligo.
    b. Chloasma.
    c. Acrodynia.
    d. Freckle.

18. The vitiligo in this location is resistant to typical treatments for cutaneous vitiligo due to the lack of hair follicles and melanocytes'?
    a. vitiligo on hand.
    b. Labial Mucosa vitiligo.
    c. Vitiligo on facial skin.
    d. Vitiligo on the chin.

19. The following pigmented disorder can occur in patients undergoing immunotherapy to treat Malignant Melanoma?
    a. Albinism.
    b. Vitiligo.
    c. Chloasma.
    d. Acrodynia.

20. The drug that causes melanosis by forming drug complexes or chelates when used to treat acne?
    a. Minocycline.
    b. Amoxicillin.
    c. Erythromycin.
    d. Ampicillin.

21. The characteristic bronzing of the skin occurs in the following disorder?
    a. Haemochromatosis.
    b. Acrodynia.
    c. Carotenemia.
    d. Melasma.

22. The blue-grey or purple pigmentation caused by gold therapy in the treatment of Rheumatoid arthritis?
    a. Chrysiasis.
    b. Acrodynia.
    c. Carotenemia.
    d. Haemochromatosis.

23. A non-invasive, in-vivo technique of inspection of pigmented skin lesions helped by a magnifier with an inbuilt illumination system that assesses the structures deep to the depth of reticular dermis, used to differentiation of suspicious melanocytic lesions from dysplastic lesions and melanomas, keratinocyte skin cancers like Basal cell carcinoma, Squamous cell carcinoma and can record images for future comparison is called?
    a. Epiluminescence microscopy.
    b. Trichoscopy.
    c. Gonioscopy.
    d. Onychoscopy.
24. The term "Erythroplasia of Queyrat" refers to red demarcated plaques affecting the?
    a. Carcinoma of Buccal Mucosa.
    b. Carcinoma-in situ of Glans Penis.
    c. Carcinoma of Labial Mucosa.
    d. Carcinoma of vermilion border of Lip.

25. The intraoral site for melanoma is?
    a. Hard Palate.
    b. Buccal Mucosa.
    c. Alveolar Mucosa.
    d. Gingiva.

26. The yellow-orange pigmentation of skin caused by excess carotene levels in blood does not affect?
    a. Oral Mucous Membrane.
    b. Facial skin.
    c. Skin of the abdomen.
    d. Skin of the forearm.

27. The characteristic appearance of Moon facies, diffuse mucocutaneous hyperpigmentation, weight Gain is a feature of the following disease?
    a. Cushing's disease.
    b. Freckle.
    c. Melasma.
    d. Chrysiasis.

28. The topical bleaching creams contain the following?
    a. Azelaic acid or 4% Hydroquinone.
    b. Azelastine.
    c. Azithromycin.
    d. Allopurinol.

29. The cause of hyperpigmentation in immune dysregulation with HIV / AIDS is increased melanin synthesis by the following hormone?
    a. α-MSH from anterior Pituitary.
    b. GH.
    c. LH.
    b. FSH.

30. Punch grafting is beneficial in the treatment of following pigmented disorder?
    a. Vitiligo.
    b. Melasma.
    c. Freckle.
    d. Chyrsiasis.

31. The extravasated blood after trauma initially appears bright red, later turn brown due to the following biochemical change?
    a. Degradation of transferrin to iron.
    b. Degradation of iron to transferrin.
    c. Degradation of iron to Hemosiderin.
    d. Degradation of Hemosiderin to iron.

Answers

1. d. Tyrosine.
2. a. Nevi.
3. a. Compound Naevi.
4. a. Blue Naevi.
5. b. Borders regular.
6. a. Clarks.
7. a. Breslow.
8. d. Nodular Melanoma.
9. a. Nevus of Ota.
10. a. Nevus of Ito.
11. a. Pulsed Q-Switched Alexandrite Laser. (755 nm, 100ns).
12. c. Icterus.
13. a. Von Recklinghausen's Disease.
14. c. Amalgam tattoo.
15. b. Silver.
16. a. Chloasma.
17. a. Vitiligo.
18. b. Labial mucosa vitiligo.
19. b. Vitiligo.
20. a. Minocycline.
21. a. Haemochromatosis.
22. a. Chrysiasis.
23. a. Epiluminescence microscopy.
24. b. Carcinoma-in situ of Glans Penis.
25. a. Hard Palate.
26. a. Oral mucous membrane.
27. a. Cushing's disease.
28. a. Azelaic acid or 4% Hydroquinone.
29. a. α-MSH from anterior Pituitary.
30. a. Vitiligo.
31. c. Degradation of iron to Haemosiderin.

Chapter 5

SARS-CoV-2

Questions

1. Severe Acute Respiratory Syndrome Coronavirus 2 (SARS-CoV-2) is a?
   a. Single-stranded RNA Virus
   b. Double-stranded DNA Virus
   c. Single-stranded DNA Virus
   d. Double-stranded RNA Virus

2. SARS-Cov -2 belongs to the family of the following viruses?
   a. Alpha coronaviruses
   b. Beta coronaviruses
   c. Gamma coronaviruses
   d. Delta corona viruses

3. SARS-Cov-2 belongs to the member of the subgenus of the following virus?
   a. Sarbeco virus
   b. Adenovirus
   c. Entero virus
   d. Hetero virus

4. The viral envelope in SARS-Cov -2 is constituted by these proteins EXCEPT?
   a. Spike Protein
   b. Envelope Protein
   c. Nucleocapsid Protein
   d. Membrane Protein

5. The spike protein can be imaged at the atomic level by what microscopy?
   a. Cryogenic electron Microscopy
   b. Ultraviolet Microscopy
   c. Electron Microscopy
   d. Microscopy

6. The protein in SARS-Cov -2 responsible for allowing the virus to attach to and fuse with the Host cell membrane is?
   a. Spike protein
   b. Membrane protein.
   c. Nucleocapsid Protein
   d. Core Protein.

7. SARS-CoV-2 has sufficient affinity to the receptor on human cells?
   a. Angiotensin-converting enzyme (ACE-1)
   b. Angiotensin-converting enzyme (ACE-2)
   c. Angiotensin-converting enzyme (ACE-3)
   d. Angiotensin-converting enzyme (ACE-4)

8. The painful, itchy, red patches on the extremities caused by cold exposure and tend to ulcerate in covid-19 patients?
   a. Chilblains
   b. Cold Sores
   c. Frostbite
   d. Bite mark

9. The following therapy is beneficial in treating covid patients?
   a. Convalescent plasma therapy
   b. Iontophoresis
   c. Dialysis
   d. Bemer therapy

10. The most common anticoagulant implicated in binding to covid-19 spike protein and causes downregulation of Interleukin-6?
    a. Low molecular weight Heparin
    b. Clopidrogel
    c. Dipyridamole
    d. Digabatrin

Answers

1. a. Single-stranded RNA Virus.
2. b. Beta coronavirus.
3. a. Sarbeco virus.
4. a. Spike Protein.
5. a. Cryogenic Electron Microscopy.
6. a. Spike Protein.
7. b. Angiotensin-converting Enzyme- 2.
8. a. Chilblains.
9. a. Convalescent plasma therapy.
10. a. Low molecular weight Heparin.

Chapter 6

Ulcerative Lesions of the Oral Cavity

Questions

1. The ulcer caused by the tongue rasping against newly erupted Primary incisors is called?
   a. Behcet's ulcer
   b. Eosinophilic ulcer
   c. Riga Fede ulcer
   d. Tuberculous ulcer

2. These ulcers occur solitary?
   a. Aphthous ulcer
   b. Eosinophilic ulcer
   c. Traumatic ulcer
   d. Behcet's disease

3. Can the following clinically present as an ulcer on the Palate?
   a. Aphthous ulcer
   b. Mucormycosis
   c. Riga-fede ulcer
   d. Eosinophilic ulcer

4. The following disease can cause ulcers, often in areas of trauma, commonly on the buccal mucosa along the occlusal plane?
   a. Pemphigus Vulgaris
   b. Aphthous ulcer
   c. Traumatic ulcer
   d. Eosinophilic ulcer

5. A lace-like ulcer characterizes the following disease with a purulent surface on a red base with a granular or cobblestone appearance?
   a. Pemphigus Vulgaris
   b. Pemphigus vegetans
   c. Pemphigus foliaceus
   d. Pemphigus erythematosus

6. The ulcer that occurs as a complication of severe burns due to acute gastric erosion?
    a. Curling's ulcer
    b. Riga fede ulcer
    c. Eosinophilic ulcer
    d. Aphthous ulcer

7. Immune-mediated disorders, EXCEPT, cause the following ulcer?
    a. Traumatic ulcer
    b. Aphthous ulcer
    c. Erythema multiforme
    d. Extranodal NK-T cell Lymphoma

8. The ulcer caused by following illicit drugs, except?
    a. Cocaine
    b. Amphetamine
    c. Methylenedioxymethamphetamine (MDMA)
    d. Tramadol

9. An ulcer caused by a neglected tropical disease caused by Mycobacterium ulcerans?
    a. Buruli ulcer
    b. Martorell's ulcer
    c. Cushing's ulcer
    d. Rodent ulcer

10. The ulcer caused by the malignant transformation of chronic wounds?
    a. Marjoulin's ulcer
    b. Martorell's ulcer
    c. Cushing's ulcer
    d. Rodent ulcer

11. The ulcer that occurs near the nasolabial fold and can burrow?
    a. Martorell's ulcer
    b. Marjoulin's ulcer
    c. Rodent ulcer
    d. Cushing's ulcer

12. The ulcer caused by poorly controlled systemic hypertension?
    a. Martorell's ulcer
    b. Marjoulin's ulcer
    c. Rodent ulcer
    d. Cushing's ulcer

Answers

1. c. Riga Fede Ulcer.
2. c. Traumatic Ulcer.
3. b. Mucormycosis.
4. a. Pemphigus Vulgaris.
5. b. Pemphigus Vegetans.
6. a. Curling's ulcer.
7. a. Traumatic Ulcer.
8. d. Tramadol.
9. a. Buruli ulcer.
10. a. Marjoulin's ulcer.
11. c. Rodent ulcer.
12. a. Martorell's ulcer.

Chapter 7

Vesiculobullous Disorders Affecting the Oral Cavity

Questions

1. The following autoantibodies are formed against the following in Pemphigus?
    a. Epithelium
    b. Connective tissue
    c. Intercellular adhesion substance Desmoglein
    d. Basement membrane

2. The fibrinous adhesions of the palpebral conjunctiva to the sclera restricting eyeball movement are called?
    a. Symblepharon
    b. Ptosis
    c. Entropion
    d. Trichiasis

3. The inwardly placed eyelashes in patients affected by cicatricial pemphigoid are called?
    a. Ectropion
    b. Entropion
    c. Symblepharon
    d. Trichiasis

4. The inwardly placed eyelashes injuring the cornea causing corneal injury or ulcer is called?
    a. Ectropion
    b. Entropion
    c. Symblepharon
    d. Trichiasis

5. The best transport medium for samples suspected of Vesiculobullous lesion is?
    a. Mitchell's solution
    b. Saline
    c. Dextrose
    d. Mannose

6. Which of the following intercellular surface glycoprotein in oral epithelium affected in patients with Pemphigus?
   a. Desomglein 1
   b. Desmoglein 2
   c. Desmoglein 3
   d. Desmoglein 4

7. The standard Gold method for diagnosis of Paraneoplastic Pemphigus is?
   a. Immunoprecipitation
   b. Periodic acid Schiff stain
   c. Asboe-Hansen sign
   d. Nikolsy's sign

8. The gingival involvement of this vesiculobullous disorder mimic desquamative Gingivitis?
   a. Cicatricial Pemphigoid
   b. Lichen planus
   c. Bullous Pemphigoid
   d. Epidermolysis Bullosa Dystrophica

9. Paraneoplastic Pemphigus is seen among patients with the following disorder?
   a. Myeloproliferative disorders
   b. Lymphoproliferative disorders
   c. Melanoma
   d. Sarcoma

10. The earliest change in Mucous membrane Pemphigoid is?
    a. Subconjunctival Fibrosis
    b. Corneal ulcer
    c. Haemmorhagic Crusting of Lips
    d. Outwardly placed eyelashes

11. The term "cicatricial" in Cicatricial Pemphigoid refers to?
    a. Erosion
    b. Vesicle
    c. Ulcer
    d. Scar

12. The vesiculobullous disorder associated with microstomia, reduced depth of the labial vestibule, mitten-like deformity of hand due to repeated trauma and scarring is?
    a. Epidermolysis Bullosa Dystrophica
    b. Pemphigus Vulgaris
    c. Cicatricial Pemphigoid
    d. Paraneoplastic Pemphigus

13. Thc carliest changes in gingiva is seen in the following vesiculobullous disorder?
    a. Pemphigus Vulgaris
    b. Epidermolysis Bullosa Dystrophica
    c. Cicatricial Pemphigoid
    d. Bullous lichen planus

14. The Pemiphigus lesions are differentiated from Pemphigoid lesions by the following signs and symptoms?
    a. Easily rupturable Bullae
    b. Tense thick-walled Bullae
    c. Conjunctival scar
    d. Symblepharon

15. The drug implicated in causing Pemphigus?
    a. Captopril
    b. Enalapril
    c. Perindropril
    d. Lisinopril

16. The drug used to relieve joint pain and swelling in Rheumatoid arthritis but can lead to Pemphigus?
    a. Prednisolone
    b. Beclomethasone
    c. Penicillamine
    d. Methylprednisolone

17. Paraneoplastic tic Pemphigus can have the highest incidence among the following Malignancies?
    a. Non-Hodgkin's Disease
    b. Hodgkin's Disease
    c. Sarcoma
    d. Thymoma

18. The auto-antigens targeted in Paraneoplastic Pemphigus?
    a. Envoplakin and Periplakin
    b. Desmoglein 1
    c. Desmoglein 3
    d. Bullous Pemphigoid antigen

Answers

1. c. Intercellular adhesion substance Desmoglein.
2. a. Symblepharon.
3. b. Entropion.
4. d. Trichiasis.
5. a. Mitchell's solution.
6. c. Desmoglein-3.
7. a. Immunoprecipitation.
8. a. Cicatricial Pemphigoid.
9. b. Lymphoproliferative disorders.
10. a. Subconjunctival fibrosis.
11. d. Scar.
12. a. Epidermolysis bullosa dystrophica.
13. a. Pemphigus Vulgaris.
14. a. Easily rupturable Bullae.
15. a. Captopril.
16. c. Penicillamine.
17. d. Thymoma.
18. a. Envoplakin and Periplakinn.

Chapter 8

Bacterial Infections of the Oral Cavity

Questions

1. The Bacteria that commonly colonizes Human Mouth?
   a. Actinomycosis.
   b. Poxvirus.
   c. Rabies virus.
   d. Poliovirus.

2. The term for disseminated tuberculosis spread through the bloodstream with lesions resembling millet seeds?
   a. Miliary Tuberculosis.
   b. Lumpy Jaw syndrome.
   c. Reactivation Tuberculosis.
   d. Primary Tuberculosis.

3. The primary tuberculosis lesions are confined to the middle portion of the lungs, called?
   a. Miliary Tuberculosis.
   b. Ghon's complex.
   c. Lumpy jaw.
   d. Whitlow.

4. The Tuberculous infection of the spine is called?
   a. Ghon's complex.
   b. Whitlow.
   c. Pott's disease.
   d. Leonine.

5. The Mantoux test is considered positive if induration is more than, following injection of 0.1 ml of purified protein derivative?
   a. 10 mm.
   b. 15 mm.
   c. 20 mm.
   d. 25 mm.

6. What is the vegetative growth of the internal organs such as the liver and spleen resulting in Hepatomegaly and splenomegaly caused by Bartonella henselae?
   a. Pleiosis.
   b. Mitosis.
   c. Meiosis.
   d. Anisocytosis.

7. Amber coloured encrustations of the perioral skin and vermilion border is seen in the following?
   a. Erysipelas.
   b. Impetigo.
   c. Pleiosis.
   d. Diptheria.

8. In immunocompromised patients, the extensive blackish orofacial necrosis of the cheek occurs in?
   a. Noma.
   b. Impetigo.
   c. Pleiosis.
   d. Erysipelas.

9. The following bacterial infection can also produce sulphur granules and mimic actinomycosis?
   a. Botryomycosis.
   b. Coccidiomycosis.
   c. Histoplasmosis.
   d. Mucormycosis.

10. Conjunctivitis or conjunctival granuloma associated with preauricular lymphadenopathy transmitted by rubbing the eye after grooming the cat's skin is called?
    a. Oculoglandular syndrome of Parinaud.
    b. Histoplasmosis.
    c. Actinomycosis.
    d. Botryomycosis.

Answers

1. a. Actinomycosis.
2. a. Miliary Tuberculosis.
3. b. Ghon's complex.
4. c. Pott's disease.
5. b. 15 mm.
6. a. Pleiosis.
7. b. Impetigo.
8. a. Noma.
9. a. Botryomycosis.
10. a. Oculoglandular syndrome of Parinaud.

Chapter 9

Viral Infections of the Oral Cavity

1. The virus with a long replicating cycle?
   a. Herpes simplex I.
   b. Herpes simplex II.
   c. Varicella-zoster.
   d. Cytomegalo virus.

2. The virus that causes Fatal Encephalitis?
   a. Hepatitis B virus.
   b. Cytomegalo virus.
   c. Epstein- Barr virus.
   d. Varicella zoster virus.

3. The unique characteristic of Latent infection is seen in the family of these viruses?
   a. Herpes virus.
   b. Poxvirus.
   c. Poliovirus.
   d. Rubeola virus.

4. The virus that induces no cytopathic changes in the cell culture systems?
   a. Epstein Barr Virus.
   b. Poxvirus.
   c. Rubella virus.
   d. Cytomegalovirus.

5. Does the herpes simplex virus replicate in the following cell?
   a. Epithelial cells.
   b. Muscle cells.
   c. Myoepithelial cells.
   d. Melanotic cells.

6. Which of the following are referred to as "cold sores" as lesions caused by which virus?
   a. Recurrent Herpes simplex type I virus.
   b. Recurrent Pox virus.
   c. Recurrent cytomegalovirus.
   d. Recurrent Epstein Barr virus.

7. Herpes simplex virus infection in abraded skin of fingers among health care workers is called?
   a. Herpetic whitlow.
   b. Herpes Gladiatorum.
   c. Cold sores.
   d. Hot spot.

8. Herpes simplex Encephalitis is characterised by haemorrhagic necrosis of the inferior-medial portion of which lobe?
   a. Occipital Lobe.
   b. Temporal Lobe.
   c. Parietal Lobe.
   d. Frontal Lobe.

9. Which of the following, the replication of cytomegalovirus, is most prominent?
   a. Salivary Glands.
   b. Brain.
   c. Muscle.
   d. Heart.

10. The virus associated with Kaposi sarcoma?
    a. HHV-6
    b. HHV-7
    c. HHV-8
    d. HHV-9

11. What is the Zoonotic virus that fruit bats of Pteropopidae family can transmit?
    a. Poliovirus.
    b. Herpes Zoster virus.
    c. Nipah Virus.
    d. Retrovirus.

12. The virus that results in Microcephaly and other neurological complications in Pregnant women?
    a. Zika virus.
    b. Nipah virus.
    c. Poliovirus.
    d. Herpes zoster virus.

13. The infection of the following virus causes Burkitt's Lymphoma?
    a. Ebstein Barr virus.
    b. Poliovirus.
    c. Nipah virus.
    d. Zika virus.

14. Epstein Barr virus is implicated in the following pathogenesis, EXCEPT?
    a. Burkitt's Lymphoma.
    b. Erythema Multiforme.
    c. Infectious Mononucleosis.
    d. Bacillary angiomatosis.

15. The Zoonotic virus Nipah virus belongs to the family and genus?
    a. Paramyxoviridae; Henipavirus.
    b. Herpes viridae; Lymphocrypto virus.
    c. Retro virus; Lenti virus.
    d. Herpesviridae; simplex virus.

16. The Epstein Barr virus belongs to the family and genus?
    a. Retrovirus; Lentivirus.
    b. Herpesviridae; Lymphocrypto virus.
    c. Paramyxoviridae; Henipavirus.
    d. Paramyxo virus; Henipavirus.

17. The Human Immunodeficiency Virus (HIV) belongs to the family and genus?
    a. Paramyxo virus; Lymphocrytpto virus.
    b. Retrovirus; Lentivirus.
    c. Herpes viridae; Lymphocrypto virus.
    d. Herpesviridae; Simplex virus.

Answers

1. d. Cytomegalo virus.
2. a. Hepatitis B virus.
3. a. Herpes virus.
4. a. Ebstein barr virus.
5. a. Epithelial cells.
6. a. Recurrent Herpes Simplex Type I Virus.
7. a. Herpetic whitlow.
8. b. Temporal Lobe.
9. a. Salivary glands
10. c. HHV-8.
11. c. Nipah virus.
12. a. Zika virus.
13. a. Ebstein Barr virus.
14. d. Bacillary angiomatosis.
15. a. Paramyxoviridae; Henipa virus.
16. b. Herpesviridae; Lymphocrypto virus.
17. b. Retro virus; Lenti virus.

Chapter 10

Fungal Infections of the Oral Cavity

Questions

1. The diagnostic test for deep invasive candidiasis is?
   a. β-D Glucan Assay
   b. α-D Glucan Assay
   c. γ-D Glucan Assay
   d. α-L-Glucan Assay

2. The assay based on detecting antibodies against the surfaces of c. albicans germ tubes by indirect immunofluorescence?
   a. CAGTA (Candida Albicans Germ Tube Assay)
   b. GTA (Germ Tube Assay)
   c. TA (Tube Assay)
   d. TACG (Tube Assay candidiasis Germ Tube)

3. The assay specific for the diagnosis of invasive aspergillosis?
   a. Galactomannan Assay (GM)
   b. GTA (Germ Tube Assay)
   c. TA (Tube Assay)
   d. CAGTA (Candida Albicans Germ Tube Assay)

4. The diagnostic tool that assesses volatile organic compounds in patients with invasive aspergillosis?
   a. E-noses (Electronic Noses).
   b. Halimeter
   c. Breathalyser
   d. Gastrolyzer

5. The drug of choice for prevention and salvage therapy of fungal infections in adults?
   a. Posoconazole
   b. Itraconazole
   c. Fluconazole
   d. Miconazole

6. The volatile metabolites of Aspergillus fumigatus include?
   a. α and β- trans -bergamotene or trans-geranylacetone.
   b. Γ trans-bergamotene
   c. α- trans-geranylacetone
   d. γ-trans-bergamotene

7. The fungus associated with rotting vegetation proliferates at an elevated temperature greater than 40 degrees Celsius?
   a. Aspergillus
   b. Candidiasis
   c. Mucormycosis
   d. cryptococcus

8. The Aspergillosis fungus can cause an abscess in the brain, which looks like a?
   a. Cannonball
   b. Tennis ball
   c. Cricket ball
   d. Ball in hand

9. The small round encapsulated yeast cells seen by analysing Cerebrospinal fluid after Indian ink preparations?
   a. Cryptococcus
   b. Candidiasis
   c. Aspergillus
   d. Mucormycosis

10. The reverse-halo or inversed halo or atoll sign is a characteristic finding in patients in Computed Tomography imaging of lung in patients affected?
    a. Mucormycosis
    b. Aspergillosis
    c. Candidiasis
    d. Cryptococcosis

11. The European Society of Clinical Microbiology and Infectious Diseases Fungal Infection Study Group (ESCMID) and European Confederation of Medical Microbiology recommends the following for the treatment for Mucormycosis?
    a. i.v Liposomal Amphotericin 5mg/kg body weight
    b. i.v Liposomal Amphotericin 4 mg/kg body weight
    c. i.v Liposomal Amphotericin 3 mg/kg body weight
    d. i.v Liposomal Amphotericin 2 mg/ kg body weight

12. The diagnosis of candida esophagitis is?
    a. single contrast esophagography
    b. Double-contrast esophagography
    c. Unicontrast esophagography
    d. Bi-contrast esophagography

13. Candida esophagitis is best delineated by double-contrast esophagography, which characteristically appears as the following after barium swallow?
    a. Feather appearance
    b. Ball appearance
    c. Cotton fluffy appearance
    d. Circular appearance

14. The following number of lung lesions characterise invasive pulmonary aspergillosis?
    a. 10 Pulmonary nodules and Pleural effusion
    b. 5 Pulmonary nodules and Emphysema
    c. 15 Pulmonary nodules and Empyema
    d. 3 Pulmonary nodules and Pleural effusion

Answers

1. a. β-D Glucan assay.
2. a. CAGTA (Candida Albicans Germ Tube Assay).
3. a. Galactomannon Assay.
4. a. E-Noses (Electronic Noses).
5. a. Posoconazole.
6. a. α and β- trans -bergamotene or trans-geranylacetone
7. c. Mucormycosis.
8. a. Cannon Ball.
9. a. Cryptococcosis.
10. a. Mucormycosis.
11. a. i.v Liposomal Amphotericin 5mg/kg body weight.
12. b. Double contrast esophagography.
13. a. Feather appearance.
14. b. 5 Pulmonary nodules and Emphysema.

Chapter 11

Temporomandibular Joint Disorders

Questions

1. The length of the condyle in an adult range from approximately?
   a. 20mm mediolaterally, 8-10mm anteroposteriorly
   b. 10 mm mediolaterally, 5-7mm anteroposteriorly
   c. 30 mm mediolaterally, 10-12 mm anteroposteriorly
   d. 40 mm mediolaterally, 6-8 mm anteroposteriorly

2. Complete calcification of the cortical borders in a TMJ may not be completed by the following year?
   a. Five years of age
   b. Ten years of age
   c. Fifteen years of age
   d. Twenty years of age

3. The medial pole of the condylar neck is angled with the sagittal plane by the following angulation?
   a. 10-20 degrees
   b. 15-33 degrees
   c. 10-15 degrees
   d. 20-30 degrees

4. Does the articular eminence develop during the following years of age?
   a. First 2 years of age
   b. First 3 years of age
   c. First 4 years of age
   d. First 5 years of age

5. Pneumatization of articular eminence is seen radiographically in approximately the following percentage of patients?
   a. 1%
   b. 2%
   c. 3%
   d. 4%

6. The source of pain in cases of internal derangement of TMJ, when the posterior attachment becomes trapped between the condyle and articular eminence is?
   a. Retrodiscal tissues
   b. Bilaminar zone
   c. Anterior band
   d. Posterior band

7. The superior lamina component that helps stretch and allow the articular disc to move forward with condylar translation and then allows for the smooth recoil of the disc posteriorly during mandibular closure is?
   a. Fibrin
   b. Laminin
   c. Elastin
   d. Actin

8. The shape of the articular disc?
   a. Biconcave
   b. Biconvex
   c. Convex
   d. Concave

9. The Posterior band of the articular disc sits at the superior aspect of the condyle in the following clock position?
   a. 9 '0' clock position
   b. 10 '0' clock position
   c. 11 '0' clock position
   d. 12 '0' clock position

10. The retrodiscal tissues, as the condyle move forward, they expand in volume because of the following distension?
    a. Arterial distension
    b. Venous distension
    c. Capillary distension
    d. Mechanical distension

11. The following part is the source of pain in the anterior disc displacement of internal derangement?
    a. Retrodiscal tissues
    b. Anterior band thick
    c. Bilaminar venous plexus
    d. Posterior extension

12. Inferior condylar positioning is seen in the following, EXCEPT?
    a. Blood within the joint space
    b. Fluid within joint space
    c. Effusions within joint space
    d. Perforations of the articular disc

13. Superior condylar positioning is seen, EXCEPT?
    a. Displacement of the articular disc
    b. Perforation of the articular disc
    c. Fluid within Joint space
    d. Loss of attachment of the articular disc

14. The condyle found within a range of posterior to the crest of articular eminence?
    a. 1-2 mm
    b. 2-3mm
    c. 2-5mm
    d. 2-6mm

15. The condyle is seen within a range of anterior to the crest of articular eminence?
    a. 3-4mm
    b. 4-5mm
    c. 5-6 mm
    d. 5-8mm

16. Hypermobility of TMJ may be suspected if the condyle translates more than 5mm anterior to the eminence?
    a. 3mm
    b. 4mm
    c. 5mm
    d. 6mm

17. The following image sequences in MRI demonstrate the osseous and discal tissues of TMJ?
    a. T1 weighted images
    b. T2 weighted images
    c. Proton weighted images
    d. Diffusion-weighted images

18. The following image sequences in MRI demonstrate the inflammation and joint effusion of TMJ?
    a. T1-weighted images
    b. T2-weighted images
    c. Proton weighted images
    d. Diffusion-weighted images

19. The growth centre for mandible?
    a. Condylar cartilage
    b. Hyaline cartilage
    c. Fibro-cartilage
    d. Coronoid process

20. The form of hyperplastic condyle varies from the following shape?
    a. Spherical
    b. Conical
    c. shortened
    d. Elongated

21. Can condylar hyperplasia be differentiated from a condylar osteoma or large osteophyte in degenerative joint disease?
    a. In condylar hyperplasia, both right and left sides of TMJ are affected
    b. In condylar osteoma, both right and left sides of TMJ are affected
    c. In Degenerative Joint disease osteoarthritis, both right and left sides of TMJ are affected
    d. Osteophytes, both right and left sides of TMJ, are affected

22. Is the undersized mandibular condyle that may result from congenital, developmental, or acquired diseases that affect condylar growth?
    a. Condylar Hypoplasia
    b. Condylar Hyperplasia
    c. Bifid condyle
    d. Toadstool condyle

23. The term Boering's arthrosis refers to?
    a. Juvenile arthrosis
    b. Osteoarthritis
    c. Rheumatoid arthritis
    d. Gonococcal arthritis

24. The pseudo-Joint that may develop between the hyperplastic coronoid process and the posterior surface of the zygoma is called?
    a. Max joseph space
    b. Boering's arthritis
    c. Superior joint space
    d. Jacob's disease

25. Coronoid hyperplasia, the tip of the coronoid process must at least extend above the following distance from the inferior rim of the zygomatic arch?
    a. 1 cm
    b. 2 cm
    c. 3 cm
    d. 4 cm

26. The following characteristic shape of the condyle is seen in patients with bifid condyle?
    e. Heart-shaped
    f. Cone-shaped
    g. Flattening of condyle
    h. Toadstool condyle

27. The articular disc of the Temporomandibular Joint is usually displaced in the following direction?
    a. Anterior
    b. Posterior
    c. Superior
    d. Inferior

28. The following imaging modality is a gold standard in imaging the articular disc of TMJ?
    a. OPG
    b. CT
    c. MRI
    d. CBCT

29. In sagittal sections of MRI, the articular disc appears like the shape?
    a. Bow tie
    b. Cone
    c. Elongated
    d. Reduced

30. The expected direction of displacement of the articular disc?
    a. Anterior displacement
    b. Posterior displacement
    c. Superior displacement
    d. Inferior displacement

31. Perforations in the articular disc commonly occur in these parts of the articular disc of the Tempero mandibular Joint?
    a. Anterior band
    b. Posterior band
    c. Intermediate zone
    d. Retro discal tissue

32. The best investigation for detecting Perforations in the articular disc is?
    a. Computed Tomography
    b. Magnetic Resonance Imaging
    c. Arthrography
    d. Arthroplasty

33. What are the masses of fibrous tissue or scar tissue that form in the Temporomandibular joint space after TMJ surgery?
    a. Fibrous adhesions
    b. Perforations
    c. Internal derangement
    d. Degenerative Arthritis

34. The phenomenon of "struck disc" in which the normal movement of the articular disc is restricted is seen in the following Temporomandibular disorder?
    a. Perforations
    b. Internal derangement
    c. Fibrous adhesions
    d. Degenerative arthritis

35. The adaptive response of cartilage and skeletal tissue to forces applied to the Joint that may be excessive, resulting in alteration in the shape of the condyle and articular eminence is called?
    a. Remodelling
    b. Perforation
    c. Fibrous Adhesions
    d. Degenerative arthritis

36. The remodelling changes in the Temporomandibular Joint involve all these changes, EXCEPT?
    a. Flattening
    b. Thickening of the cortex of articulating surfaces
    c. Subchondral sclerosis
    d. Decreases the number of trabeculations resulting in reduced density

37. The non-inflammatory joint disorder characterized by both deterioration and bony proliferation?
    a. Remodelling
    b. Ostcoarthritis
    c. Perforation
    d. Fibrous adhesions

38. The areas of degeneration containing small, round radiolucent areas with irregular margins with regions of increased bone density in degenerative joint disease are called?
    a. Ely's cysts
    b. Perforation
    c. Remodelling
    d. Fibrous adhesions

39. The projections of new bone formed at the articular surfaces in degenerative joint disease are called?
    a. Osteophyte
    b. Osteocyte
    c. Osteoclast
    d. Osteoblast

40. Osteophytes, EXCEPT cause the following?
    a. Usually create broader, flatter articular surfaces
    b. Extend from articular eminence to encase the condylar head
    c. Can break off and lie free within Joint space
    d. Do not break off

41. The characteristic imaging findings of the following TMJ disorder result from villous synovitis, which helps form granulomatous synovial tissue (Pannus) that grows into fibrocartilage and bone releasing enzymes that destroy the articular surfaces and underlying bone?
    a. Rheumatoid arthritis
    b. Osteoarthritis
    c. Degenerative joint disease
    d. Psoriatic arthritis

42. Decreased Temporomandibular Joint function can lead to following changes in bone?
    a. Decrease in the number of trabeculations resulting in decreased density
    b. Increase in the number of trabeculations and decreased density
    c. Do not either increase the number of trabeculations and density
    d. Increase in the number of trabeculations and increased density

43. A non-inflammatory disorder affecting the Temporomandibular Joint?
    a. Rheumatoid arthritis
    b. Psoriatic arthritis
    c. Osteoarthritis
    d. Gonococcal arthritis

44. The subchondral pseudocysts located within the temporomandibular Joint containing osteoid, granulation tissue is called?
    a. Ely's cysts
    b. Stafne cyst
    c. Dentigerous cyst
    d. Radicular cyst

45. The bone spur is also called?
    a. Osteophyte
    b. Blastocyte
    c. Pericyte
    d. Chondrocyte

46. Which of the following are true about osteophytes, EXCEPT?
    a. Can also grow in the spine
    b. Limit movement
    c. can cause pain and stiffness of the joint
    d. Do not break off

47. Bouttoniere deformity of the thumb and swan-neck deformity of fingers is seen in following arthritis?
    a. Rheumatoid arthritis
    b. Osteoarthritis
    c. Gonococcal arthritis
    d. Psoriatic arthritis

Answers

1. a. 20mm mediolaterally, 8-10mm anteroposteriorly.
2. d. 2O years of age.
3. b. 15-33 degrees.
4. c. First 4 years of age.
5. b. 2%
6. a. Retrodiscal Tissues.
7. c. Elastin.
8. a. Biconcave.
9. c. 11 'O" Clock Position.
10. b. Venous Distension.
11. b. Retrodiscal Tissues.
12. d. Perforations of the articular disc.
13. c. Fluid within joint space.
14. c. 2-5 mm.
15. d. 5-8 mm.
16. c. 5mm.
17. c. Proton weighted images.
18. b. T2 weighted images.
19. a. Condylar Cartilage.
20. c. Shortened.
21. a. In condylar hyperplasia, both right and left sides of TMJ are affected.
22. a. Condylar Hypoplasia.
23. a. Juvenile arthrosis.
24. d. Jacob's disease.
25. a. 1 cm.
26. a. Heart-shaped.
27. a. Anterior.
28. c. MRI.
29. a. Bow tie.
30. a. Anterior Displacement.
31. d. Retrodiscal tissue.
32. c. Arthrography.
33. a. Fibrous adhesions.
34. c. Fibrous adhesions.
35. a. Remodelling.
36. d. Decreases the number of trabeculations resulting in decreased density.
37. b. Osteoarthritis.
38. a. Ely's cysts.

39. a. Osteophyte.
40. d. Do not break off.
41. a. Rheumatoid arthritis.
42. a. Decrease in the number of trabeculations resulting in decreased density.
43. c. Osteoarthritis.
44. a. Ely's cysts.
45. a. Osteophyte.
46. d. Do not break off.
47. a. Rheumatoid arthritis.

Chapter 12

Diseases of the Maxillary Sinus

Questions

1. The largest of all Paranasal sinus in humans is?
   a. Frontal sinus
   b. Ethmoid sinus
   c. Maxillary sinus
   d. Sphenoid sinus

2. The membranous lining of the maxillary sinus is called?
   a. Schneiderian membrane
   b. Transitional
   c. Tight junction
   d. Fibrinous adhesions

3. The most anterior ethmoidal cells lying anterolateral and inferior to the frontal recess and anterior and above the attachment of the middle turbinate and are within the lacrimal bone and therefore have as lateral relations the orbit, the lacrimal sac and the nasolacrimal duct, may contribute to frontal sinusitis?
   a. Agger nasi
   b. Haller cells
   c. Columnar cells.
   d. Cuboidal cells.

4. The infraorbital ethmoidal air cells located lateral to the maxillo-ethmoidal suture along the inferior-medial orbital floor?
   a. Haller cells
   b. Agger nasi
   c. Cuboidal cells.
   d. Tzanck cells.

5. The posterior-most ethmoidal air cell extends posteriorly to lie superolateral to the sphenoid sinus and thus near the optic nerve and internal carotid artery?
   a. Onodi cell
   b. Haller cells
   c. Agger nasi
   d. Supraorbital air cell.

6. A benign, self-limiting disease caused by leakage of mucus within the sinus mucosa due to ductal obstruction resulting in a convex soft tissue mass within the maxillary sinus on Computed Tomography imaging?
   a. Mucous retention cyst of Maxillary sinus
   b. Maxillary sinusitis
   c. Acute Maxillary sinusitis
   d. Maxillary Osteomyelitis

7. The first sinus to develop in the maxillofacial complex and mimic the symptoms of odontogenic origin?
   a. Ethmoid sinus.
   b. Maxillary sinus.
   c. Frontal sinus.
   d. Sphenoid sinus.

8. The Maxillary sinus develops during the following intrauterine life?
   a. First month of Intrauterine Life.
   b. Second month of intrauterine Life.
   c. Third Month of Intrauterine Life.
   b. Fourth month of Intrauterine Life.

9. The phenomenon can be confused with benign space-occupying lesions in plain extraoral projections?
   a. Pneumatization.
   b. Spallation.
   c. Amplification.
   d. Stimulation.

10. The thickness of a normal sinus mucosa is?
    a. 1mm.
    b. 2 mm.
    c. 3 mm.
    d. 4 mm.

11. During inflammation, the sinus can increase in thickness, of the normal?
    a. 5-10 mm.
    b. 10-15 mm.
    c. 15-20 mm.
    d. 20-25 mm.

12. The term used to denote sinuses involving the Maxillofacial complex is called?
    a. Pansinusitis.
    b. Acute sinusitis.
    c. Chronic sinusitis.
    d. Subacute sinusitis.

13. The following is not associated with periapical disease?
    a. Mucous retention Pseudocyst.
    b. Acute Maxillary sinusitis.
    c. Polyps.
    d. Chronic Maxillary sinusitis.

14. The following can destroy the bone?
    a. Maxillary sinusitis.
    b. Polyps.
    c. Mucous retention pseudocyst.
    d. Pan sinusitis.

15. The following disease can cause ipsilateral proptosis due to the destruction of Lamina Papyracea?
    a. Frontal sinus.
    b. Maxillary sinus.
    c. Ethmoid sinus.
    d. Sphenoid sinus.

16. The most common neoplasm affecting the paranasal sinuses?
    a. Squamous cell carcinoma.
    b. Osteomas.
    c. Squamous Papilloma.
    d. Lymphomas.

17. The following do not cause obliteration of the Maxillary sinus?
    a. Paget's disease.
    b. Ossifying fibromas.
    c. Fibrous dysplasia.
    d. Maxillary sinusitis.

18. The term for pus containing Mucocele is also called?
    a. MucoPyocele.
    b. Mucocele.
    c. Cephalocele.
    d. Encephalocele.

19. The diplopia and proptosis can occur by extending the following into the orbit?
    a. Antral Polyps.
    b. Maxillary sinusitis.
    c. Mucous retention cyst and osteomas of the Maxillary sinus.
    d. Paget's disease.

20. The following disorder can cause displacement and reduce the size of the Maxillary sinus?
    a. Antral Polyps.
    b. Maxillary sinusitis.
    c. Fibrous dysplasia.
    d. Paget's disease.

Answers

1. c. Maxillary sinus.
2. a. Schneiderian membrane.
3. a. Agger nasi.
4. a. Haller cells.
5. a. Onodi cells.
6. a. Mucous retention cyst of the Maxillary sinus.
7. b. Maxillary sinus.
8. b. Second month of intrauterine life.
9. a. Pneumatization.
10. a. 1mm.
11. b. 10-15 mm.
12. a. Pansinusitis.
13. a. Mucous retention Pseudocyst.
14. b. Polyps.
15. c. Ethmoid sinus.
16. a. Squamous cell carcinoma.
17. a. Paget's Disease.
18. a. Mucopyocele.
19. c. Mucous retention cysts and osteomas of the Maxillary sinus.
20. c. Fibrous dysplasia.

Chapter 13

Cysts of the Oral and Maxillofacial Region

Questions

1. The Radicular cyst that results from stimulation of the following in the periodontal ligament?
   a. Reduced enamel epithelium.
   b. Stellate reticulum.
   c. Enamel organ.
   d. Epithelial cell rests of Malassez.

2. The most common location of radicular cysts are?
   a. Maxillary incisors and canines.
   b. Maxillary Premolars and molars.
   c. Maxillary canine and Premolars.
   d. Mandibular incisors and Molars.

3. The following dimension of radiolucency is characteristic of cyst?
   a. 0.5 cm.
   b. 1 cm.
   c. 2 cm.
   d. 2 cm.

4. The cyst that occurs when a tooth infected by radicular cyst is extracted, but cyst remains?
   a. Radicular cyst.
   b. Residual cyst.
   c. Dentigerous cyst.
   d. Odontogenic keratocyst.

5. The Dentigerous cyst is more likely if the follicular space is more than the following dimension?
   a. 3mm.
   b. 4 mm.
   c. 5 mm.
   d. 6 mm.

6. The Dentigerous cyst, if chronically infected, can transform into the following tumour?
   a. Ameloblastoma and Squamous cell carcinoma.
   b. Squamous cell carcinoma and Mucoepidermoid carcinoma.
   c. Ameloblastoma and Mucoepidermoid carcinoma.
   d. Clear cell carcinoma and Squamous cell carcinoma.

7. The most common location for Buccal bifurcation cyst is?
   a. Maxillary first molar.
   b. Mandibular first molar.
   c. Maxillary canine.
   d. Mandibular canine.

8. The epicentre for Buccal bifurcation cyst is?
   a. above crown of tooth.
   b. Periapical region of the tooth.
   c. Bifurcation region of the tooth.
   d. Crestal alveolar ridge area.

9. Satellite microcysts occurs in the lining of the following cyst?
   a. Radicular cyst.
   b. Odontogenic keratocyst.
   c. Buccal bifurcation cyst.
   d. Dentigerous cyst.

10. The epicentre of odontogenic keratocyst lies?
    a. Inferior to the inferior alveolar canal.
    b. Superior to the inferior alveolar canal.
    c. Above the crown of the tooth.
    d. Bifurcation region of roots.

11. The epithelial lining of the following cyst has got an innate growth potential?
    a. Radicular cyst.
    b. Dentigerous cyst.
    c. Odontogenic Keratocyst.
    d. Lateral Periodontal cyst.

12. Considerable expansion of odontogenic keratocyst occurs in the following regions?
    a. Coronoid process and upper ramus.
    b. Condylar process and lower ramus.
    c. Symphyses and ramus of the mandible.
    d. Parasymphyseal region of the mandible.

13. The colour of the aspirate obtained from odontogenic keratocyst is?
    a. Straw coloured.
    b. Viscous Honey coloured.
    c. Viscous cheesy.
    d. Viscous chocolate coloured.

14. The following cyst tends to grow along the internal aspect of the jaws, causing minimal expansion of the cortical plates?
    a. Radicular cyst.
    b. Odontogenic keratocyst.
    c. Dentigerous cyst.
    d. Buccal bifurcation cyst.

15. The cyst that can occur as multiple small cysts from epithelial rests in periodontium lateral to the tooth root is?
    a. Botyroid odontogenic cyst.
    b. Radicular cyst.
    c. Odontogenic keratocyst.
    d. Dentigerous cyst.

16. The cyst, when secondarily infected, can mimic lateral Periodontal abscess?
    a. Radicular cyst.
    b. Lateral Periodontal cyst.
    c. Odontogenic keratocyst.
    d. Dentigerous cyst.

17. The cyst that can mimic small ameloblastoma?
    a. Radicular cyst.
    b. Odontogenic keratocyst.
    c. Botyroid odontogenic cyst.
    d. Dentigerous cyst.

18. The rare cyst derived from odontogenic epithelium with characteristics of mucus-producing cells and hypothesized to have a relationship with mucoepidermoid carcinoma?
    a. Radicular cyst.
    b. Odontogenic keratocyst.
    c. Glandular odontogenic cyst.
    d. Dentigerous cyst.

19. The following cyst's internal structure shows small foci of calcified material that appear as white specks or small smooth pebbles or large, solid, amorphous masses due to the propensity to form dysplastic dentin or associated with odontoma?
    a. Radicular cyst.
    b. Gorlin's cyst.
    c. Dentigerous cyst.
    d. Odontogenic keratocyst.

20. The cyst that occurs as a slight, well-defined swelling with palatine papilla?
    a. Nasopalatine duct cyst.
    b. Radicular cyst.
    c. Dentigerous cyst.
    d. Odontogenic keratocyst.

21. The cyst that causes posterior bowing of the nasal fossa in Computed Tomography scan?
    a. Radicular cyst.
    b. Dentigerous cyst.
    c. Nasolabial cyst.
    d. Nasopalatine duct cyst.

22. The cyst that can simulate an acute dentoalveolar abscess?
    a. Nasolabial cyst.
    b. Lateral Periodontal cyst.
    c. Odontogenic keratocyst.
    d. Botyroid odontogenic cyst.

23. The most common congenital cyst occurs in the midline as a slow-growing painless mass at the level of or below the hyoid bone or above the hyoid bone to the tongue.
    a. Thyroglossal cyst.
    b. Radicular cyst.
    c. Lateral Periodontal cyst.
    d. Dentigerous cyst.

24. The cyst that can occur as a slow-growing painless fluctuant swelling on the lateral aspect of the neck anterior to sternocleidomastoid muscle?
    a. Thyroglossal cyst.
    b. Dermoid cyst.
    c. Branchial cleft cyst.
    d. Lateral Periodontal cyst.

25. The cyst that manifest clinically as an enlargement of the parotid gland, related to human immunodeficiency virus infections and histologically resemble Branchial cleft cyst?
    a. Dermoid cyst.
    b. Lymphoepithelial cyst.
    c. Lateral Periodontal cyst.
    d. Odontogenic keratocyst.

26. A cystic form of a teratoma thought to be derived from trapped totipotent embryonic cells?
    a. Thyroglossal cyst.
    b. Branchial cleft cyst.
    c. Dermoid cyst.
    d. Radicular cyst.

27. Which cyst often occur inside Fibrous dysplasia lesions and Cemento-osseous dysplasia?
    a. Simple bone cyst.
    b. Radicular cyst.
    c. Calcifying odontogenic cyst.
    d. Glandular odontogenic cyst.

28. The cyst that often scallops between the teeth' roots and is discovered by chance during radiological examinations?
    a. Radicular cyst.
    b. Simple bone cyst.
    c. Calcifying odontogenic cyst.
    d. Dentigerous cyst.

Answers

1. d. Epithelial Cell rests of Malassez.
2. a. Maxillary incisors and canines.
3. d. >2 cm.
4. b. Residual cyst.
5. c. 5 mm.
6. b. Squamous cell carcinoma and Mucoepidermoid carcinoma.
7. b. Mandibular First Molar.
8. c. Bifurcation region of the teeth.
9. b. Odontogenic Keratocyst.
10. b. Superior to inferior alveolar canal.
11. c. Odontogenic Keratocyst.
12. a. Coronoid Process and Upper Ramus.
13. c. Viscous cheesy.
14. b. Odontogenic Keratocyst.
15. a. Botyroid odontogenic cyst.
16. b. Lateral Periodontal cyst.
17. c. Botyroid odontogenic cyst.
18. c. Glandular Odontogenic cyst.
19. b. Gorlin's cyst.
20. a. Nasopalatine duct cyst.
21. c. Nasolabial cyst.
22. a. Nasolabial cyst.
23. a. Thyroglossal cyst.
24. c. Branchial cleft cyst.
25. b. Lymphoepithelial cyst.
26. c. Dermoid cyst.
27. a. Simple Bone cyst.
28. b. Simple Bone cyst.

Chapter 14

Odontogenic Tumors

Questions

Benign Tumours

1. The following are the characteristics of a benign tumour except?
   a. Resemble the tissue of origin histologically.
   b. Slow-growing.
   c. Spread by Direct extension.
   d. Metastases.

2. An intraosseous epithelial odontogenic tumour locally invasive, anatomically benign, and clinically persistent?
   a. Ameloblastoma.
   b. Odontogenic keratocyst.
   c. Calcifying epithelial odontogenic tumour.
   d. Cementoblastoma.

3. The tumours that produce a mineralized substance within amyloid-like material contain strands or sheets of polyhedral cells in fibrous stroma?
   a. Calcifying Epithelial odontogenic Tumor.
   b. Ameloblastoma.
   c. Adenomatoid odontogenic Tumor.
   d. Ameloblastic fibro odontoma.

4. The Benign mixed odontogenic tumour formed by neoplastic proliferation of odontogenic epithelium and primitive mesenchymal components resembling the Dental Papilla?
   a. Calcifying Epithelial odontogenic Tumor.
   b. Adenomatoid odontogenic Tumor.
   c. Ameloblastic fibroma.
   d. Ameloblastoma.

5. The odontogenic tumour with an enamel-like or dentinoid material?
   a. Ameloblastoma.
   b. Calcifying Epithelial odontogenic Tumor.
   c. Adenomatoid odontogenic tumor.
   d. Ameloblastic fibroma.

6. A rare, benign mesenchymal tumour that resembles the mesenchymal portion of dental papilla has straight internal septa?
   a. Ameloblastoma.
   b. Myxoma.
   c. Calcifying Epithelial Odontogenic Tumor.
   d. Odontoma.

7. The tumour of neuroectodermal origin arising from Schwann cells makes up the inner layer covering the peripheral nerves is?
   a. Ameloblastoma.
   b. Neurilemmoma.
   c. Odontoma.
   d. Myxoma.

8. The Codman triangle occurs in the following tumour?
   a. Odontoma.
   b. Neurilemmoma.
   c. Osteosarcoma.
   d. Myxoma.

9. An abnormal communication between an artery and vein bypassing the intervening capillary bed due to trauma or development and extraction of the associated tooth can cause life-threatening bleeding?
   a. Arterio-venous aneurysm.
   b. Odontoma.
   c. Ameloblastoma.
   d. Osteoblastoma.

10. An aggressive form of ossifying fibroma occurs within the first two years of life?
    a. Ossifying fibroma.
    b. Osteoid osteoma.
    c. Osteoblastoma.
    d. Cementoblastoma.

11. An odontogenic tumour that can arise secondarily in tissues that have received therapeutic levels of radiation?
    a. Fibrosarcoma.
    b. Osteosarcoma.
    c. Ewing sarcoma.
    d. ossifying fibroma.

12. A tumour that arises from the medullary portion of the bone spreads to the endosteal and later periosteal surface of the bone, which can mimic symptoms of sinusitis and associated trismus?
    a. Osteosarcoma.
    b. Ewing sarcoma.
    c. Ossifying fibroma.
    d. Osteoid osteoma.

13. The tumour with the propensity to grow along with the soft tissue spaces (fatty areas) and the surface of the bone?
    a. Osteosarcoma.
    b. Ewing sarcoma.
    c. Non-Hodgkin's Lymphoma.
    d. Ossifying fibroma.

14. The tumour that rarely produces a reactive bone within its centre appears radiolucent in radiographs is?
    a. Burkitt's Lymphoma.
    b. Ewing sarcoma.
    c. Non-Hodgkin's Lymphoma.
    d. Osteosarcoma.

15. The tumour with the propensity to grow in the Periodontal ligament space of well-developed mature teeth?
    a. Non-Hodgkin's Lymphoma.
    b. Ewing sarcoma.
    c. Burkitt's Lymphoma.
    d. Osteosarcoma.

Answers

1. d. Metastases.
2. a. Ameloblastoma.
3. a. Calcifying epithelial odontogenic tumour.
4. c. Ameloblastic fibroma.
5. c. Adenomatoid odontogenic tumour.
6. b. Myxoma.
7. b. Neurilemmoma.
8. c. Osteosarcoma.
9. a. Arterio-venous aneurysm.
10. a. Ossifying fibroma.
11. a. Fibrosarcoma.
12. b. Ewing sarcoma.
13. c. Non-Hodgkin's Lymphoma.
14. a. Burkitt's Lymphoma.
15. a. Non-hodgkin's Lymphoma.

Chapter 15

Osteodystrophies and Diseases of the Bone

Questions

1. The term used to denote a localized change in normal bone metabolism that replaces all the cancellous bone components by fibrous tissue containing varying amounts of abnormally appearing woven bone?
   a. Fibrous dysplasia.
   b. Osteosclerosis.
   c. Condensing osteitis.
   d. Rarefying osteitis.

2. Fibrous dysplasia results from a mutation in the following gene in a chromosome?
   a. Gs alpha (GNAS1 gene) on chromosome 20q13.32
   b. Gs Beta (GNAS2 gene) on chromosome 21 q 13.33
   c. Gs Gamma (GNAS3 gene) on chromosome 22 q 13.34
   d. Gs Delta (GNAS4 gene) on chromosome 23 q 13.35.

3. The Craniofacial fibrous dysplasia can impinge on the nerve foramina resulting in these complications, EXCEPT?
   a. Anosmia.
   b. Deafness.
   c. Blindness.
   d. Tardive dyskinesia.

4. The characteristic radiological feature of Fibrous dysplasia is?
   a. Shattered windshield appearance.
   b. Spider-web appearance.
   c. Honey-comb appearance.
   d. Cart-wheel appearance.

5. The characteristic of Fibrous dysplasia is its organization of abnormal trabeculae into a swirling pattern similar to a?
   a. The skin of an orange.
   b. Fingerprint.
   c. Honeycomb.
   d. Cartwheel.

6. Extension of Fibrous dysplasia into the Maxillary antrum usually results from the following direction?
   a. Medial wall.
   b. Lateral wall.
   c. Floor.
   d. Apex.

7. The last section of the Maxillary sinus to be involved from Fibrous dysplasia predominantly is?
   a. Most Anteroposterior location.
   b. Most Posterosuperior portion.
   c. Most superoinferior portion.
   d. Most Antero inferior location.

8. The lesions of Fibrous dysplasia are unique in that they can displace the inferior alveolar canal in a?
   a. Inferior direction.
   b. Superior direction.
   c. Anterior direction.
   d. Posterior direction.

9. Which of these lesions can occur within the lesions of Fibrous dysplasia?
   a. Dentigerous cyst, Aneurysmal bone cyst.
   b. Aneurysmal bone cyst; Giant cell Granuloma.
   c. Dentigerous cyst; Ameloblastoma.
   d. Aneurysmal bone cyst; Ameloblastoma.

10. The most common site of occurrence of Periapical osseous dysplasia is?
    a. Maxillary anterior.
    b. Mandibular anterior.
    c. Maxillary molars.
    d. Mandibular molars.

11. A bone disease in which the normal cancellous bone is replaced with dense, acellular amorphous bone compromises blood supply and likely contributes to infection?

    a. Florid Cemento-osseous dysplasia.
    b. Periapical osseous dysplasia.
    c. Fibrous dysplasia.
    d. Peripheral ossifying fibroma.

12. A skeletal disorder involving osteoclasts resulting in abnormal resorption and apposition of osseous tissues poor in quality in one or more bones?
    a. Fibrous dysplasia.
    b. Periapical osseous dysplasia.
    c. Paget's disease.
    d. Florid Cementoosseous dysplasia.

13. Patients with Paget's disease may have ill-defined neurological pain due to the?
    a. Bone impingement on nerve canals and foramina.
    b. Non-bone impingement on nerve canals and foramina.
    c. Enlargement of the skull.
    d. Malocclusion of teeth.

14. Patients with Paget's disease have the following in urine?
    a. Proline.
    b. Hydroxyproline.
    c. Lysine.
    d. Hydroxylysine.

15. The trabeculae in Paget's disease gets arranged in these patterns during the early, intermediate and late appositional stages of bone deposition, EXCEPT?
    a. Radiolucent.
    b. Granular or Ground Glass appearance.
    c. More radiopaque cotton wool-like appearance.
    d. Sunburst appearance.

16. The incidence of jaw osteomyelitis is higher in the following bone disorder?
    a. Paget's Disease.
    b. Fibrous Dysplasia.
    c. Periapical osseous dysplasia.
    d. Osteosclerosis.

17. Paget's disease is managed medically by all, EXCEPT?
    a. Calcitonin.
    b. Sodium etidronate.
    c. Bisphosphonates.
    d. Steroids.

18. The epicentre of bone destruction in Langerhans cell Histiocytosis is approximately in the following region of the tooth?
    a. Cervical root region.
    b. Mid root region.
    c. Apical root region.
    d. Cemento enamel junction region.

Answers

1. a. Fibrous Dysplasia.
2. a. Gs alpha (GNAS1 gene) on chromosome 20q13.32
3. d. Tardive Dyskinesia.
4. a. Shattered Windshield appearance.
5. b. Finger Print Pattern.
6. b. Lateral Wall.
7. b. Most Postero Superior Location.
8. b. Superior Direction.
9. b. Aneurysmal Bone cyst; Giant cell Granuloma.
10. b. Mandibular anterior.
11. a. Florid Cemento-osseous Dysplasia.
12. c. Paget's Disease.
13. a. Bone impingement on Nerve canals and Foramina.
14. b. Hydroxy Proline.
15. d. Sun Burst appearance.
16. a. Paget's Disease.
17. d. Steroids.
18. b. Midroot region.

Chapter 16

Disorders of Teeth

Questions

1. The teeth that develop morphologically normal or abnormal besides the usual complement because of excess dental lamina in the jaws is called?
   a. Supernumerary teeth.
   b. Dilaceration.
   c. Concrescence.
   d. Fusion.

2. The missing teeth in the jaws due to the absence of one or few teeth is called?
   a. Hyperdontia.
   b. Hypodontia.
   c. Supernumerary teeth.
   d. Supplementary teeth.

3. The condition in which all the teeth fail to develop?
   a. Hyperdontia.
   b. Hypodontia.
   c. Oligodontia.
   d. Anodontia.

4. The most common missing teeth are?
   a. Maxillary third molars.
   b. Maxillary incisors.
   c. Maxillary Premolars.
   d. Maxillary first molars.

5. The term used to denote larger-sized teeth than usual is?
   a. Microdontia.
   b. Macrodontia.
   c. Hyperdontia.
   d. Oligodontia.

6. The difference between Fusion and Gemination is that?
    a. The count of teeth reveals a missing tooth in Fusion.
    b. The count of teeth does not reveal a missing tooth in Fusion.
    c. The count of teeth does not reveal a missing tooth in Gemination.
    d. Clinical evidence of either cleft in crown or root of teeth is present in Fusion.

7. The term used for a condition in which two adjacent teeth have exchanged positions in the dental arch is called?
    a. Transposition.
    b. Fusion.
    c. Gemination.
    d. Concrescence.

8. The most frequently transposed teeth are?
    a. Permanent incisor and Premolars.
    b. Permanent Lateral incisor and central incisors.
    c. Permanent canine and first Premolars.
    d. Permanent mandibular premolars and molars.

9. The term used to denote Fusion of teeth that results from the union of adjacent tooth germs of developing teeth?
    a. Hypodontia.
    b. Oligodontia.
    c. Synodontia.
    d. Hyperdontia.

10. The term used to denote when the roots of two or more primary or permanent teeth are fused by cementum?
    a. Fusion.
    b. Concrescence.
    c. Synodontia.
    d. Hyperdontia.

11. The tooth anomaly arises when a single tooth bud attempts to divide, resulting in invagination of the crown with partial division or complete division resulting in two identical structures?
    a. Fusion.
    b. Gemination.
    c. Concrescence.
    d. Twinning.

12. The common area affected by Twinning?
    a. Permanent incisor region.
    b. Primary incisor region.
    c. Permanent Premolar region.
    d. Permanent molar region.

13. The peculiar radiological feature of Taurodontism is?
    a. Foreshortened Pulp chamber and more coronally positioned furcation.
    b. Elongated Pulp chamber and more coronally positioned furcation.
    c. The elongated pulp chamber and more apically positioned furcation.
    d. Foreshortened Pulp chamber and more apically positioned furcation.

14. Which of the following tooth anomaly have a "Bull's eye appearance"?
    a. Fusion Labially or Lingually.
    b. Gemination Mesially or Distally.
    c. Dilaceration Labially or Lingually.
    d. Concrescence -mesially or distally.

15. The term "tooth within a tooth" is indicated for the following dental anomaly?
    a. Dens in dente.
    b. Gemination.
    c. Fusion.
    d. Concrescence.

16. The radicular variety of Dens invaginatus usually affects these teeth?
    a. Mandibular first premolars and second molars.
    b. Maxillary first premolars and second molars.
    c. Maxillary incisors and canines.
    d. Mandibular incisors and canines.

17. Dens invaginatus and dens in dente occur in the tooth in the following order of decreased frequency?
    a. Permanent maxillary lateral incisors > Maxillary central incisors > Maxillary Premolars > Maxillary canines > Maxillary molars.
    b. Permanent maxillary lateral incisors < Maxillary central incisors < Maxillary Premolars < Maxillary canines < Maxillary molars.
    c. Permanent Maxillary central incisor < Maxillary Premolars < Maxillary molars < Maxillary canine < Maxillary canine.
    d. Permanent Maxillary central incisor > Maxillary Premolars > Maxillary molars > Maxillary canine > Maxillary canine.

18. The dental anomaly that results from an outpouching of enamel organ is?
    a. Dens invaginatus.
    b. Dens in dente.
    c. Dens evaginatus.
    d. Fusion.

19. The most commonly affected teeth by Dens evaginatus are?
    a. Maxillary central incisors.
    b. Maxillary Lateral incisors.
    c. Mandibular central incisors.
    d. Mandibular Lateral incisors.

20. The Amelogenesis Imperfecta, which is most easily identifiable on imaging?
    a. Hypoplastic type.
    b. Hypomaturation type.
    c. Hypocalcification.
    d. Hypomaturation with Taurodontism.

21. The snowcapped appearance is seen in the following Amelogenesis imperfecta?
    a. Hypoplastic.
    b. Hypomaturation.
    c. Hypocalcification.
    d. Hypomaturation with Taurodontism.

22. The characteristic appearance of anterior teeth in Amelogenesis imperfecta is?
    a. Picket fence appearance.
    b. Mulberry appearance.
    c. Tooth within a tooth appearance.
    d. Triangular appearance.

23. A rare dental anomaly in which both the enamel and dentin are hypoplastic and hypocalcified?
    a. Regional odontodysplasia.
    b. Amelogenesis imperfecta.
    c. Dentinogenesis imperfecta.
    d. Taurodontism.

24. The teeth affected by Type I Dentin dysplasia are associated with rarefying osteitis because?
    a. Microscopic communication between the oral cavity and residual pulp.
    b. Absence of communication between the oral cavity and residual pulp.
    c. Lack of communication between residual pulp and dentin.
    d. Communication between residual pulp and dentin.

25. The shape of the molar roots in Type I Dentin dysplasia is?
    a. U shape.
    b. V Shape.
    c. W shape.
    d. X shape.

26. The teeth affected by Regional Odontodysplasia have the following characteristic appearance?
    a. Ghost-like appearance.
    b. Picket fence appearance.
    c. Tooth within a tooth appearance.
    d. Globular appearance.

27. A small spherical mass of enamel measuring 1-3 mm in diameter at the bifurcation region of molars is called?
    a. Enamel drop.
    b. Dens evaginatus.
    c. Dens invaginatus.
    d. Dilated Odontome.

28. Enamel drops are typical among the furcal areas of posterior teeth?
    a. Mesial or distal Furca of Maxillary molars; Buccal and Lingual Furca in Mandibular molars.
    b. Buccal or Lingual Furca of Maxillary Molars; Mesial and Distal Furca in Mandibular molars.
    c. Buccal and Lingual Furca of Maxillary molars.
    d. Mesial and Distal Furca of Mandibular molars.

29. The dental anomaly resulting from extension of periapical infection from its deciduous predecessor or mechanical trauma transmitted through the deciduous tooth?
    a. Talon cusp.
    b. Turners Hypoplasia.
    c. Dens evaginatus.
    d. Dens invaginatus.

30. The teeth affected most commonly by Turner's Hypoplasia?
    a. Maxillary incisors.
    b. Mandibular canines.
    c. Mandibular Premolars.
    d. Mandibular molars.

31. In congenital syphilis, Hutchinson's incisor, do the Maxillary central incisors have a characteristic shape?
    a. Screw driver shape.
    b. Cone shaped.
    c. Picket fence shape.
    d. Globular shape.

32. The molars in congenital syphilis have the following characteristic shape: the enamel formed over the occlusal surface in irregular globules called?
    a. Mulberry.
    b. Pear shaped.
    c. Cone shaped.
    d. Squarish.

33. The improper "back and forth" movements of the toothbrush with heavy pressure cause the bristles to form a wedge-shaped arrangement between teeth and gingiva, resulting in the following shaped groove near the cervical area of the tooth?
    a. "V" Shape.
    b. "W" Shape.
    c. "X" shape.
    d. "Y "shape.

34. The most common location for Abrasion is?
    a. Maxillary molars.
    b. Maxillary canine.
    c. Maxillary Premolars.
    d. Maxillary incisors.

35. The areas of cervical erosion can be differentiated from cervical Abrasion?
    a. Cervical erosion appears more rounded off than cervical Abrasion.
    b. Cervical Abrasion appears more rounded off than cervical erosion.
    c. Cervical erosion results in a V-shaped defect.
    d. Cervical abrasion results in a semilunar-shaped defect.

36. External resorption of the tooth is due to these causes, EXCEPT?
    a. Excessive function.
    b. Odontogenic cysts and tumors cause excess pressure.
    c. Chronic inflammation.
    d. Direct or indirect Pulp capping.

37. The following are the causes for Internal tooth resorption, EXCEPT?
    a. Acute trauma to teeth.
    b. Pulpotomy.
    c. Direct and Indirect Pulp capping.
    d. Dentin invagination.

38. The teeth most commonly affected by Internal resorption are?
    a. Permanent maxillary central incisors, first and second molars.
    b. Permanent maxillary lateral incisors, first and second molars.
    c. Permanent maxillary premolars, first and second molars.
    d. Permanent maxillary canine, first and second molars.

39. The internal resorption can be differentiated from caries on the buccal or lingual surface of the tooth?
    a. The image of internal resorption cannot be separated from the pulp chamber or canal by altering the horizontal angulation of the beam.
    b. The image of internal resorption can be separated from the pulp chamber or canal by altering the vertical angulation of the beam.
    c. The image of internal resorption cannot be separated from the pulp chamber or canal by altering the vertical angulation of the beam.
    d. The image of internal resorption can be separated from the pulp chamber or canal by altering the horizontal angulation of the beam.

40. Dutch cheese molars are the soft, porous discolored enamel in the first permanent molars?
    a. Molar incisor Hypomineralization.
    b. Amelogenesis imperfecta.
    c. Dentino genesis imperfecta.
    d. Dental fluorosis.

41. The following drug therapy group is implicated as a cause for molar-incisor Hypomineralization in children younger than five years?
    a. Analgesics.
    b. Non-steroidal anti-inflammatory drugs.
    c. Anti-fungal drugs.
    d. Ani-neoplastic therapy.

42. The rate of apposition of Deciduous enamel is estimated?
    a. 0.013 mm/day.
    b. 0.023 mm/day.
    c. 0.033 mm/day.
    d. 0.043 mm/day.

43. The intrinsic discoloration of teeth due to the deposition of Porphyrins in the teeth?
    a. Gunther's disease.
    b. Ochronosis.
    c. Chlorodontia.
    d. Dental fluorosis.

44. Which of the deposition cause the greenish discoloration of teeth in addition to enamel hypoplasia?
    a. Stercobilin.
    b. Bilirubin.
    c. Biliverdin.
    d. Stercobilinogen.

Answers

1. a. Supernumerary Teeth.
2. b. Hypodontia.
3. d. Anodontia.
4. a. Maxillary Third Molars.
5. b. Macrodontia.
6. a. The count of teeth reveals a missing tooth in Fusion.
7. a. Transposition.
8. c. Permanent canine and First Premolars.
9. c. Synodontia.
10. b. Concrescence.
11. d. Twinning.
12. b. Primary incisor region.
13. c. Elongated Pulp chamber and apically positioned furcation.
14. c. Dilaceration-Labially or Lingually.
15. a. Dens in Dente.
16. a. Mandibular first Premolars and second molars.
17. a. Permanent maxillary lateral incisors > Maxillary central incisors> Maxillary Premolars> Maxillary canines> Maxillary molars.
18. c. Dens evaginatus.
19. b. Maxillary Lateral incisors.
20. a. Hypoplastic type.
21. b. Hypomaturation.
22. a. Picket fence appearance.
23. a. Regional odontodysplasia.
24. a. Microscopic communication between the oral cavity and residual pulp.
25. c. W shape.
26. a. Ghost-like appearance.
27. a. Enamel drop.
28. a. Mesial or distal furca of Maxillary molars; Buccal and Lingual furca in Mandibular molars.
29. b. Turners Hypoplasia.
30. c. Mandibular Premolars.
31. a. Screwdriver shape.
32. a. Mulberry.
33. a. “V “Shape.
34. c. Maxillary Premolars.
35. a. Cervical erosion appears more rounded off than cervical abrasion.
36. d. Direct or Indirect Pulp capping.
37. d. Dentin invagination.
38. a. Permanent maxillary central incisors, first and second molars.
39. a. The image of internal resorption cannot be separated from the pulp chamber or canal by altering the horizontal angulation of the beam.
40. a. Molar incisor Hypomineralization.

41. d. Anti-neoplastic therapy.
42. b. 0.023 mm/ day.
43. a. Gunther's disease.
44. c. Biliverdin.

Chapter 17

Diseases of Pulp

Questions

1. The term used to denote the condition in which the microbial products of inflammation are attracted towards the area of inflammation?
   a. Anachoretic Pulpitis.
   b. Acute Pulpitis.
   c. Chronic Pulpitis.
   d. Transient Pulpitis.

2. The nodular calcified masses that occur within the coronal pulp chamber?
   a. Pulp Polyp.
   b. Pulp stones.
   c. Pulpitis.
   d. Pulp remnants.

3. Which of the following about Pulp stones is true?
   a. Cause Pain.
   b. Cause swelling.
   c. Interfere during endodontic therapy.
   d. Do not cause pain.

4. The discrete calcifications formed during the period of root development and occur in the furcation areas of the multirooted tooth are?
   a. Pulp stones.
   b. Denticles.
   c. Diffuse Linear calcifications.
   d. Endolith.

5. The Diffuse linear calcifications are differentiated from Pulp stones?
    a. Lack of lamellar organization.
    b. Presence of Lamellar organization.
    c. Detected by Radiograph.
    d. Cause Pain and discomfort.

6. The sharp lancinating pain experienced by the patient in pulpitis is due to the involvement?
    a. A delta fibres.
    b. C fibres.
    c. D fibres.
    d. B fibres.

7. The constant dull pain in pulpitis is due to the involvement?
    a. A delta fibres.
    b. C fibres.
    c. B fibres.
    d. D fibres.

8. Increase in the intensity of pain is caused by pulpitis?
    a. Increased pulpal blood flow during recumbent position.
    b. Decreased pulpal blood flow during recumbent position.
    c. Increased pulpal blood flow during the standing position.
    d. Decreased pulpal blood flow during the standing position

9. A simple, cost-effective chair-side test for assessing pulp vitality?
    a. Thermal test.
    b. Electric pulp test.
    c. Laser Doppler flowmetry.
    d. Pulse oximetry.

10. A thermal video system with a silicon close-up lens with a resolving power of 0.023 inches that can detect temperature changes as low as 0.01°C in pulp?
    a. Hughes Probe eye camera.
    b. Electric pulp test.
    c. Pulse oximetry.
    d. Laser doppler flowmetry.

Answers

1. a. Anachoretic Pulpitis
2. b. Pulp stones.
3. d. Do not cause pain.
4. c. Diffuse Linear Calcifications.
5. a. Lack of lamellar organization.
6. a. A-delta fibers.
7. b. C fibers.
8. a. Increased Pulpal blood flow during recumbent position.
9. a. Thermal test.
10. a. Hughes Probe eye camera.

Chapter 18

Disorders of the Tongue

Questions

1. Median Rhomboid Glossitis is due to?
   a. Candidiasis.
   b. Persistence of Tuberculum impar.
   c. Lichen planus.
   d. Failure of embryonic fusion.

2. The appearance of tiny vegetative growths all over the tongue in patients with Pemphigus Vegetans is?
   a. Scrotal tongue.
   b. Magenta tongue.
   c. Strawberry tongue.
   d. Cerebriform tongue.

3. Fissured tongue is known by another name called?
   a. Scrotal Tongue.
   b. Magenta Tongue.
   c. Strawberry Tongue.
   d. Cerebriform Tongue.

4. The Sublingual varicosities are also known?
   a. Caviar Tongue.
   b. Scrotal Tongue.
   c. Cerebriform Tongue.
   d. Magenta Tongue.

5. Which of the term Saburral tongue refer?
   a. Chronic renal failure.
   b. Vitamin B 12 deficiency.
   c. Sublingual varicosities.
   d. Fissuring of the tongue.

6. The Crenated tongue is seen in the endocrine disorder?
   a. Acromegaly.
   b. Myxoedema.
   c. Secondary thyrotoxicosis.
   d. Goiter.

7. The term for describing the numerous fissures on the dorsum of the tongue?
   a. Scrotal Tongue.
   b. Saburral Tongue.
   c. Beefy red tongue.
   d. Moeller's glossitis.

8. The finger-like projections on the ventral surface of the tongue?
   a. Plica Fimbriata.
   b. Saburral tongue.
   c. Scrotal tongue.
   d. Bald tongue.

9. The Bald tongue is present in the following hematological disorder?
   a. Microcytic Hypochromic anemia.
   b. Megaloblastic macrocytic anemia.
   c. Thalassemia.
   d. Pellagra.

10. The rhythmic involuntary movements of the tongue in patients with cerebral palsy are called?
    a. Tardive dyskinesia.
    b. Bald tongue.
    c. Saburral tongue.
    d. Scrotal tongue.

Answers

1. a. Candidiasis.
2. d. Cerebriform Tongue.
3. a. Scrotal Tongue.
4. a. Caviar Tongue.
5. a. Chronic Renal Failure.
6. a. Acromegaly.
7. a. scrotal tongue.
8. a. Plica Fimbriata.
9. a. Microcytic hypochromic anemia.
10. a. Tardive dyskinesia.

Chapter 19

Disorders of Salivary Gland

Questions

1. The inflammation of the terminal duct ends in the salivary gland is?
   a. Sialadenitis.
   b. Sialosis.
   c. Sialodochitis.
   d. Sialocele.

2. The defensive enzyme in saliva?
   a. Lysozyme.
   b. Renin.
   c. Pepsin.
   d. Hydrochloric acid.

3. The non-neoplastic enlargement of the salivary gland is?
   a. Sialadenosis.
   b. Sialodochitis.
   c. Sialadenitis.
   d. Salivary adenoma.

4. The congenital absence of the salivary gland is?
   a. Aplasia.
   b. Hyperplasia.
   c. Atrophy.
   d. Hypertrophy.

5. The inflammation of the ductal system in salivary glands is?
   a. Sialodochitis.
   b. Sialadenosis.
   c. Sialadenitis.
   d. Sialosis.

6. The salivary gland disorder appears as a hot spot in the scintigraphy technique using Technetium Pertechnetate scans?
   a. Warthin's tumor.
   b. Pleomorphic adenoma.
   c. Adenoid cystic carcinoma.
   d. Mucoepidermoid carcinoma.

7. These cysts can occur within the parotid gland and are usually multicentric and reported in Patients with HIV?
   a. Benign Lymphoepithelial cysts.
   b. Sebaceous cyst.
   c. Dermoid cyst.
   d. Thyroglossal cyst.

8. The characteristic clinical feature of salivary gland swelling associated with itching is?
   a. Bacterial Sialadenitis.
   b. Viral Sialadenitis.
   c. Allergic sialadenitis.
   d. Sialadenitis secondary to sialolith.

9. The salivary component that acts as a marker in acute pancreatitis secondary to Diabetes mellitus is?
   a. Amylase.
   b. Lactoferrin.
   c. Ptyalin.
   d. Renin.

10. The transient swelling of the Parotid Gland after intubation from the General anesthetic procedure is called?
   a. Surgical Mumps.
   b. Viral Mumps.
   c. Chemical Mumps.
   d. Iodine Mumps.

11. The transient swelling of the parotid gland among percussion instrument players is?
    a. Pneumoparotid.
    b. Parotitis.
    c. Sialadenitis.
    d. Anesthetic Mumps.

12. A chronic sclerosing sialadenitis affecting the submandibular salivary gland is called?
    a. Kuttner Tumor.
    b. Warthin's Tumor.
    c. Adenoid cystic carcinoma.
    d. Oncocytoma.

13. An innovative technique performed under General or Local anesthetic procedure that uses narrow endoscopes to visualize and remove sialolith is called?
    a. Sialendoscopy.
    b. Lithotripsy.
    c. Photobiomodulation.
    d. Bemer therapy.

14. The peroral balloon surgical technique used to treat salivary duct strictures?
    a. Sialo lithotomy.
    b. Sialodochoplasty.
    c. Lithotripsy.
    d. Sialendoscopy.

15. The bacterial sialadenitis are differentiated from viral sialadenitis by theirs?
    a. Unilaterality.
    b. Bilateral involvement.
    c. Rapidity of spread.
    d. Extension into Parapharyngeal space.

Answers

1. c. Sialodochitis.
2. a. Lysozyme.
3. a. Sialadenosis.
4. a. Aplasia.
5. c. Sialadenitis.
6. b. Pleomorphic adenoma.
7. a. Benign Lymphoepithelial cysts.
8. d. Allergic sialadenitis.
9. a. Salivary amylase.
10. a. Surgical mumps.
11. a. Pneumoparotid.
12. a. Kutner tumor.
13. a. Sialendoscopy.
14. b. Sialodochoplasty.
15. a. Unilaterality.

Chapter 20

Neurological Disorders

Questions

1. A 50% decrease in blood-brain flow causes irreversible Brain injury?
   a. 1-2 minutes.
   b. 2-3 minutes.
   c. 3-4 minutes.
   d. 4-5 minutes.

2. The reversible, acute, focal neurologic deficit due to transient and localized cerebral ischemia but resulting in neurologic deficits lasting over 24 hours?
   a. Reversible ischaemic Neurological Deficit.
   b. Transient ischaemic attack.
   c. Stroke.
   d. Cerebrovascular accident.

3. Strokes that result from obstruction of the small (<5 mm diameter) penetrating arterioles supplying the basal ganglia, anterior limb of the internal capsule, less commonly cerebral white matter?
   a. Lacunar strokes.
   b. Cerebral infarction.
   c. Brainstem strokes.
   d. Pontine strokes.

4. The most specific diagnostic method for locating Stroke is?
   a. Cerebral angiography.
   b. CT.
   c. MRI.
   d. Ultrasonography.

5. The effects of Stroke on oral health include?
   a. Masticatory and Facial muscle weakness.
   b. Improved skill of arms and Hands.
   c. Dysphagia.
   d. Diminished Gag reflex.

6. Elective dental treatment must be deferred for about the following duration in a patient affected by Stroke?
   a. four months.
   b. 5 Months.
   c. 6 Months.
   d. 7 Months.

7. The characteristic plaques seen limited to white matter and Periventricular areas of CNS, Brain, spinal cord are seen?
   a. Multiple sclerosis.
   b. Stroke.
   c. Alzheimer's disease.
   d. Parkinsonism.

8. The rapid flickering contractions of the facial musculature in Multiple sclerosis patients is called?
   a. Isokymia.
   b. Myokymia.
   c. Perikymia.
   d. Retrokymia.

9. The disease, characterized by neurotic plaques and neurofibrillary tangles, which are abnormally phosphorylated tau proteins, impairs axonal transport and normal neuronal function?
   a. Multiple sclerosis.
   b. Alzheimer's disease.
   c. Stroke.
   d. Parkinsonism.

10. The Diagnostic criteria for Multiple sclerosis is?
    a. Mc Donald's criteria.
    b. Ducket Jones criteria.
    c. Sweet's criteria.
    d. Laskin's criteria.

Answers

1. c. 3-4 Minutes.
2. a. Reversible Ischaemic Neurological Deficit (RIND).
3. a. Lacunar strokes.
4. a. Cerebral Angiography.
5. b. Improved skill of arms and Hands.
6. c. 6 Months.
7. a. Multiple sclerosis.
8. b. Myokymia.
9. b. Alzheimer's disease.
10. a. Mc Donald's criteria.

Chapter 21

Haematopoietic Disorders

Questions

1. What do you mean by the term Pancytopenia?
   a. Reduction in number of RBCs, WBCS, Platelets.
   b. Reduction in Neutrophils.
   c. Reduction in Lymphocytes.
   d. Reduction in Monocytes.

2. The antifolate drug that causes an adverse effect of Macrocytic anemia?
   a. Phenytoin.
   b. Benzodiazepine.
   c. Baclofen.
   d. Hydroxyurea.

3. RBC shows many spicules due to an unstable red cell membrane lipid structure?
   a. Abetalipoproteinaemia.
   b. Paraproteinaemia.
   c. Hemolytic anemia.
   d. Myelofibrosis.

4. The fragmented RBCs sliced by fibrin bands, seen?
   a. Disseminated intravascular coagulation.
   b. Hemolytic anemia.
   c. Megaloblastic anemia.
   d. Iron deficiency anemia.

5. A marked leukocytosis (greater than 50 x 10^9 /L) seen in leukemia, burns, or infection?
   a. Leukamoid reaction.
   b. Leukocytosis.
   c. Neutrophilia.
   d. Monocytosis.

6. Irregular-shaped RBCs called Burr cells to occur in the hematological disorder?
   a. Iron deficiency anemia.
   b. Megaloblastic anemia.
   c. Thalassemia.
   d. Uraemia.

7. The RBCs with central staining and a ring of pallor and outer peripheral staining, so-called Mexican Hat cells, are seen in hematological disorder?
   a. Thalessemia.
   b. Uraemia.
   c. Paraproteinaemia.
   d. Neutropenia.

8. Ristocetin-induced platelet aggregation (RIPA) is used to diagnose?
   a. Von Willebrand's disease.
   b. Haemophilia.
   c. Eryhroblastosis foetalis.
   d. Thalassemia.

9. The sickling of red blood cells occurs due to following aminoacid substitution?
   a. Valine for Glutamate in the 6th position of Haemoglobin β chain.
   b. Glutamate for Valine in the 6th position of Haemoglobin β chain.
   c. Phenylalanine for Valine in the 6th position of Haemoglobin α chain.
   d. Valine for Phenylalanine in the 6th position of Haemoglobin α chain.

10. A rare inherited platelet disorder characterized by abnormal large-sized giant platelets?
    a. Glanzmann's thrombasthenia.
    b. May Hegglin anomaly.
    c. Thrombocytosis.
    d. Thrombocythaemia.

11. A platelet disorder characterized by defective platelet glycoprotein receptor (II b/ III a)?
    a. May Hegglin anomaly.
    b. Glanzmann's thrombasthenia.
    c. Thrombocytosis.
    d. Thrombocythaemia.

Answers

1. a. Reduction in number of RBCs, WBCs, Platelets.
2. a. Phenytoin.
3. a. Abetalipoproteinaemia.
4. a. Disseminated intravascular coagulation.
5. a. Leukamoid reaction.
6. d. Uraemia.
7. a. Thalassemia.
8. a. Von Willebrand's disease.
9. a. Valine for Glutamate in the 6th position of Haemoglobin Beta chain.
10. b. May Hegglin anomaly.
11. b. Glanzmann's thrombasthenia.

Chapter 22

Lymphoproliferative Disorders

Questions

1. Lymphomas are disorders caused by malignant proliferation of the following cell?
   a. Neutrophils.
   b. Lymphocytes.
   c. Monocytes.
   d. Basophils.

2. The characteristic mirror-image nuclei found in Hodgkin's lymphoma is?
   a. Sertoli cells.
   b. Leydig cells.
   c. Reed Sternberg cells.
   d. Oxyphilic cells.

3. The characteristic cyclical fever with long 15-28 days seen in Hodgkin's lymphoma is termed?
   a. Quartan fever.
   b. Diurnal fever.
   c. Pel-Ebstein fever.
   d. Tertian fever.

4. The staging system that influences treatment and prognosis in Hodgkin's Lymphoma is?
   a. Broader staging.
   b. Ann Arbor staging.
   c. Ducket jones criteria.
   d. McDonald's criteria.

5. The standard regimen for Hodgkin's Lymphoma is?
   a. ABVD regimen.
   b. CHOP regimen.
   c. Rituximab.
   d. Chlorambucil.

6. The lymphoproliferative disorders are derived from the following cell?
    a. T-lymphocyte.
    b. B-lymphocyte.
    c. CD8 T cells.
    d. CD4 T cells.

7. The following is a high-grade lymphoma?
    a. Follicular Lymphoma.
    b. Marginal zone lymphoma.
    c. Lymphoplasmacytoid lymphomas.
    d. Burkitt's Lymphoma.

8. The drug of choice for Large B cell Lymphomas is?
    a. CHOP regimen.
    b. ABVD regimen.
    c. CCAVP regimen.
    d. Adriamycin.

9. The drug of choice for diffuse large B cell lymphomas is?
    a. Rituximab.
    b. Vincristine.
    c. Cyclophosphamide.
    d. Dacarbazine.

10. The only form of Hodgkin's lymphoma, with a poor prognosis?
    a. Lymphocyte predominant.
    b. Lymphocyte depleted.
    c. Mixed cellularity.
    d. Nodular sclerosing.

11. Which of the following is the fastest growing tumor?
    a. Squamous cell carcinoma.
    b. Basal cell carcinoma.
    c. Burkitt's Lymphoma.
    d. Non- Hodgkin's Lymphoma.

Answers

1. b. Lymphocytes.
2. c. Reed-Sternberg cells.
3. c. Pel-Ebstein fever.
4. b. Ann Arbor staging.
5. a. ABVD regimen.
6. b. B-Lymphocyte.
7. d. Burkitt's Lymphoma.
8. a. CHOP regimen.
9. a. Rituximab.
10. b. Lymphocyte depleted.
11. c. Burkitt's Lymphoma.

Chapter 23

Myeloproliferative Disorders

Questions

1. The subsequent investigation is helpful in the diagnosis of increased red cell mass in Polycythaemia rubra vera?
   a. Radioactive Chromium (51chromium) labelled RBCs.
   b. Radioactive iodine.
   c. Radioactive Technetium Pertechnetate.
   d. Radioactive strontium.

2. The myeloproliferative disorder in which hyperplasia of megakaryocytes produces Platelet-derived growth factor, leading to intense bone marrow fibrosis and myeloid metaplasia, hemopoiesis in the spleen and liver resulting in massive splenomegaly?
   a. Polycythaemia vera.
   b. Thrombocythemia.
   c. Chronic myeloid leukemia.
   d. Myelofibrosis.

3. Characteristic Teardrop-shaped RBCs are seen in the following?
   a. Polycythaemia vera.
   b. Chronic myeloid leukemia.
   c. Myelofibrosis.
   d. Essential Thrombocythemia.

4. The Neutrophil Alkaline Phosphatase (NAP) score is decreased?
   a. Chronic myeloid leukemia.
   b. Polycythaemia vera.
   c. Myelofibrosis.
   d. Essential Thrombocythemia.

5. The Multiple Myeloma is a malignant clonal proliferation of cells?
   a. T-Lymphocyte-derived CD4 cells.
   b. Cytotoxic mediated T-lymphocytes.
   c. B lymphocytes derived Plasma cells.
   d. T-lymphocyte-derived CD8 cells.

6. The Bence Jones proteins in Multiple myeloma are?
   a. Free Ig Light chains of either kappa or lambda type.
   b. Free Ig Heavy chains of Delta type.
   c. Free Ig Heavy chains of Kappa type.
   d. Free Ig Heavy chains of lambda type.

7. The predictive test for Multiple myeloma is?
   a. β2 Microglobulin.
   b. β^2 Macroglobulin.
   c. Ceruloplasmin.
   d. Renin.
   e. Angiotensin.

8. The complications of Multiple Myeloma include the following except?
   a. Hypocalcemia.
   b. Spinal cord compression.
   c. Dialysis for acute renal failure
   d. Immunopauresis.

9. A genetic translocation between chromosomes causes chronic myeloid leukemia?
   a. Chromosomes 9 and 22.
   b. Chromosomes 10 and 23.
   c. Chromosomes 11 and 24.
   d. Chromosomes 12 and 22.

10. The International Working Group for Myelofibrosis Research and Treatment (IWG-MRT) recommended the following drug for the treatment of Myelofibrosis?
    a. Ruxolitinib.
    b. Imatinib.
    c. Bevacuzimab.
    d. Ranibizumab.

11. A CD-123 targeted agent currently approved for treating blastic plasmacytoid dendritic cell neoplasm?
    a. Tagrascofusp.
    b. Ruxolitinib.
    c. Desonumomab.
    d. Bevacuzimab.

12. The AURKA (Aurora Kinase A inhibitor) promotes megakaryocyte differentiation and helps restore atypical megakaryocytes such as the multilobed nucleus and abrogated clustering in Myelofibrosis?
    a. Alisertib.
    b. Ruxolitinib.
    c. Ranibizumab.
    d. Ibrutinib.

13. The following drug is currently approved for the treatment of anemia in Myelofibrosis patients?
    a. Alisertib.
    b. Luspatercept.
    c. Ibrutinib.
    d. Ranibizumab.

14. The drug of choice for treating thrombocytopenia in patients with Myelofibrosis?
    a. Pacritinib.
    b. Ibrutinib.
    c. Ranibizumab.
    d. Alisertib.

15. The targeted molecular therapy for managing oral submucous fibrosis helps reduce extracellular matrix by preventing phosphorylation of Transforming Growth Factor-β?
    a. Nintedanib.
    b. Ibrutinib.
    c. Ranizumab.
    d. Alisertib.

Answers

1. a. Radioactive chromium (51-chromium) labeled RBCs.
2. d. Myelofibrosis.
3. c. Myelofibrosis.
4. a. Chronic Myeloid Leukaemia.
5. c. B-lymphocyte derived Plasma cells.
6. a. Free Ig Light chains of either kappa or lambda type.
7. a. β2 Microglobulin.
8. a. Hypocalcaemia.
9. a. Chromosome 9 and 22.
10. a. Ruxolitinib.
11. a. Tagrascofusp.
12. a. Alisertib.
13. b. Luspatercept.
14. a. Pacritinib.
15. a. Nintedanib.

Chapter 24

Endocrine Disorders

Questions

1. The disorder caused by pituitary gland infarction is?
   a. cushing syndrome.
   b. Marfan syndrome.
   c. Simmond's Disease.
   d. Crohn's Disease.

2. Which of these cells causes Phaeochromocytoma?
   a. Acidophilic cells.
   b. Basophilic cells.
   c. Sertoli cells.
   d. Chromaffin cells.

3. Which of the following hormone act as a stress hormone in response to fear, flight, or fight?
   a. Epinephrine.
   b. Acidophilic cells.
   c. Basophilic cells.
   d. Leydig cells.

4. The endocrine disorder that can result from deficiency of Growth Hormone after fusion of epiphyseal plates of long bone?
   a. Acromegaly.
   b. Gigantism.
   c. Dwarfism.
   d. Cretinism.

5. Does non-pitting edema characterize the endocrine disorder due to the accumulation of myxomatous tissue in the body?
   a. Cretinism.
   b. Myxedema.
   c. Dwarfism.
   d. Gigantism.

6. The syndrome associated with ACTH insensitivity resulting in alacrimia, achalasia?
   a. Allgrove syndrome
   b. Down syndrome
   c. Mc Cune Albright syndrome
   d. Gigantism

7. Adrenal gland failure due to bleeding and massive hemorrhage into the adrenal gland caused by bacterial infection Neisseria meningitis?
   a. Down syndrome.
   b. Waterhouse-Friderichsen syndrome.
   c. Mc Cune Albright syndrome.
   d. Cretinism.

8. The deaf and mute children are seen in the following endocrine disorder?
   a. Cretinism.
   b. Gigantism.
   c. Mc Cune Albright syndrome.
   d. Acromegaly.

9. Endocrine disorder in which polyuria, polyphagia, polydipsia occur?
   a. Diabetes mellitus.
   b. Acromegaly.
   c. Phaeochromocytoma.
   d. Cushing's disease.

10. The endocrine disorder that results from lack of Antidiuretic hormone?
    a. Diabetes insipidus.
    b. Diabetes mellitus.
    c. Cushing's disease.
    d. Phaeochromocytoma.

Answers

1. c. Simmond's Disease.
2. d. Chromaffin cells.
3. a. Epinephrine.
4. a. Acromegaly.
5. b. Myxedema.
6. a. Allgrove syndrome.
7. b. Waterhouse-Friderichsen syndrome.
8. a. Cretinism.
9. a. Diabetes mellitus.
10. a. Diabetes insipidus.

Chapter 25

Orofacial Pain

Questions

1. The largest cranial nerve of the head and neck is?
   a. Facial Nerve.
   b. Trigeminal Nerve.
   c. Glossopharyngeal Nerve.
   d. Abducent nerve.

2. The following pain is also called a suicide disease?
   a. Glossopharyngeal Neuralgia.
   b. Sphenopalatine Neuralgia.
   c. Trigeminal Neuralgia.
   d. Phantom limb pain.

3. The unilateral pain associated with aura and photophobia is?
   a. Tension Headache.
   b. Cluster Headache.
   c. Migraine.
   d. Trigeminal Neuralgia.

4. The Short-lasting Unilateral Neuralgiform headache attacks with Conjunctival injection and tearing along with conjunctival lacrimation and not with rhinorrhoea is?
   a. SUNCT.
   b. Trigeminal Neuralgia.
   c. Migraine.
   d. Cluster Headache.

5. The trigeminal neuralgia with no clinically apparent neuralgic cause?
   a. Idiopathic Trigeminal neuralgia.
   b. Secondary Trigeminal neuralgia.
   c. Symptomatic Trigeminal neuralgia.
   d. Raeder Paratrigeminal neuralgia.

6. Severe Pain in and around the eye caused by lesions at the skull base associated with Horner's syndrome?
   a. Raeder Paratrigeminal neuralgia.
   b. Idiopathic trigeminal neuralgia.
   c. Secondary trigeminal neuralgia.
   d. Symptomatic trigeminal neuralgia.

7. The term refer to any pain in the head?
   a. Cephalgia.
   b. Phantom limb pain.
   c. Causalgia.
   d. Fibromyalgia.

8. The term refers to persistent burning pain in the mandible following trauma?
   a. Fibromyalgia.
   b. Causalgia.
   c. Idiopathic Trigeminal neuralgia.
   d. Raeder Paratrigeminal neuralgia.

9. A chronic facial pain without an identifiable organic disease and affects the maxilla often gets exacerbated by dental extraction?
   a. Causalgia.
   b. Atypical Facial pain.
   c. Fibromyalgia.
   d. Migraine.

10. Pain that persists for months or years after resolution of Herpes zoster rash?
    a. Postherpetic neuralgia.
    b. Migraine.
    c. Fibromyalgia.
    d. Causalgia.

Answers

1. b. Trigeminal nerve.
2. c. Trigeminal neuralgia.
3. c. Migraine.
4. a. SUNCT.
5. a. Idiopathic Trigeminal neuralgia.
6. a. Raeder Paratrigeminal neuralgia.
7. a. Cephalgia.
8. b. Causalgia.
9. b. Atypical facial pain.
10. a. Postherpetic neuralgia.

Chapter 26

Forensic Dentistry

Questions

1. The science of dentistry deals with proper handling, examination, and evaluation of dental evidence using dental radiographs, ante (before death), and postmortem (after death) photographs and DNA?
   a. Forensic dentistry
   b. Skiagraphy
   c. Pneumatography
   d. Arthrography.

2. The study of lip prints is called?
   a. Rugoscopy
   b. Cheiloscopy
   c. Bronchoscopy
   d. Endoscopy

3. The study used for the pattern of enamel rods?
   a. Cheiloscopy.
   b. Ameloglyphics.
   c. Rugoscopy.
   d. Endoscopy.

4. The study compares suspects' teeth shape, size, and position of individual teeth of suspect's dentition?
   a. Bite mark analysis
   b. cheiloscopy
   c. Dermatoscopy.
   d. Rugoscopy.

5. The study of tooth fractures resulting in the physical disruption of teeth with leaking restorations caused by barometric pressure changes caused by high altitude environment?
   a. Odontecrexis
   b. Odontoma
   c. Dense bone island
   d. Exostoses

6. Gustafson's age estimation method DOES NOT include the following Parameter?
   a. Attrition
   b. Root transparency
   c. Tertiary dentin formation
   d. Cementum apposition

7. A dental profile comprises a group of more or less specific individual characteristics relating to the oral cavity or the teeth.
   a. Dental profiling
   b. Antemortem records
   c. Photographs
   d. Infrared Photographs

8. The sorting of multiple individuals based on age and, to a lesser extent, race, and gender is called?
   a. Stratification.
   b. Gratification.
   c. Modification.
   d. Bifurcation.

9. The Primary methods used in body identification in Forensic Dentistry includes all EXCEPT?
   a. Visual identification.
   b. Fingerprint identification.
   c. Dental identification.
   d. RNA identification.

10. The following sinus morphology is variable, and this region may compare antemortem and postmortem (after death) diagnostic images for identification?
    a. Maxillary sinus.
    b. Sphenoid sinus.
    c. Ethmoid sinus.
    d. Frontal sinus.

11. The following forensic identification is of no use when the body is macerated, decomposed, or incinerated?
    a. DNA identification.
    b. Fingerprint identification.
    c. Dental identification.
    d. Visual identification.

12. The three teams formed in identification in Forensic odontology are all the following, EXCEPT?
    a. An antemortem team.
    b. Postmortem Team.
    c. A comparison team.
    d. Rescue team.

13. The following computer softwares used as an aid for comparison in Forensic sciences all EXCEPT?
    a. WinID3
    b. Plass Data.
    c. DVI system.
    d. DICOM.

14. The agencies help match the set of Human remains to a missing person EXCEPT?
    a. NamUs (National Missing and Unidentified Persons System).
    b. NCIC (National Crime Information Centre).
    c. INTERPOL.
    d. NCC.

Answers

1. a. Forensic Dentistry.
2. b. Cheiloscopy.
3. b. Ameloglyphics.
4. a. Bite Mark Analysis.
5. a. Odontocrexis.
6. c. Tertiary dentin formation.
7. a. Dental Profiling.
8. a. Stratification.
9. d. RNA identification.
10. d. Frontal sinus.
11. b. Fingerprint identification.
12. d. Rescue team.
13. d. DICOM.
14. d. NCC.

Chapter 27

Lasers in Dentistry

Questions

1. The acronym for LASER is?
   a. Light Amplification by Stimulated Emission of Radiation.
   b. Light Activated by Simulated Emission of Radiation.
   c. Light Amplified by Simultaneous Excitation of Radiation.
   d. Light Activated by Similar Excitation of Radiation

2. The first application and functioning of Laser was credited for the person named?
   a. Theodore Maiman
   b. William Harvey
   c. John miller
   d. Pateero

3. The following type of Laser has a high affinity for water?
   a. Co2
   b. Nd: YAG
   c. Erbium
   d. Diode

4. The Laser used in Laser Assisted New Attachment Procedure?
   a. Nd: YAG Laser
   b. Co2 Laser.
   c. Erbium laser
   d. Diode

5. The Laser which has a high affinity for Hydroxyapatite crystals?
   a. Nd: YAG Laser.
   b. Co2 Laser.
   c. Diode laser
   d. Erbium laser

6. The Laser helps remove inflamed and hypertrophic tissue and photostimulation of aphthous and Herpetic lesions?
   a. Diode laser.
   b. Co2 Laser.
   c. Erbium laser.
   d. Nd: YAG Laser

7. Which of the following Laser is not made up of Gaseous construction?
   a. Argon laser.
   b. Diode laser.
   c. CO2 laser.
   d. Helium-neon laser.

8. The Laser helps alter the surface chemistry of both enamel and root surface dentine, which reduces the probability of recurrent caries?
   a. Argon Laser.
   b. Co2 laser.
   c. Erbium laser.
   d. Nd: YAG Laser.

9. The Laser that is effective in cases where conventional photothermal power bleaching is not successful?
   a. KTP Laser.
   b. Co2 laser
   c. Erbium Laser.
   d. Nd: YAG Laser

10. The Laser that helps to reduce the pain associated with orthodontic force application without interfering with tooth movement?
    a. CO2 Laser.
    b. Erbium laser
    c. Nd: YAG laser.
    d. Argon laser

11. The Laser that is useful in the detection of dental caries?
    a. Argon laser (488 nm).
    b. Diode laser (633 nm).
    c. C02 Laser (10600 nm).
    d. Helium Laser (633 nm).

12. The Laser that helps to detect Pit and fissure caries by optical changes?
    a. Argon laser (488 nm).
    b. Helium-neon Laser (633 nm).
    c. Diode laser (635 nm).
    d. CO2 laser (10600 nm).

13. The Laser used in Laser Doppler flowmetry to assess pulpal blood flow?
    a. Diode laser (655 nm).
    b. Co2 Laser (10600 nm).
    c. Helium-neon laser (633 nm).
    d. Argon Laser (488 nm).

14. The Laser used for scanning Photostimulable phosphor plates in digital imaging?
    a. Helium-neon laser (633 nm).
    b. Co2 Laser (10600 nm).
    c. Argon laser (488nm).
    d. Erbium laser.

15. The Laser used in flow cytometric cell analysis?
    a. Argon laser (488 and 515 nm).
    b. CO2 Laser (10600 nm).
    c. Erbium laser.
    d. Helium-neon Laser (633 nm).

16. The Laser used in Raman spectroscopic analysis of tooth structure?
    a. Nd: YAG Laser (10600 nm).
    b. Helium-neon Laser (633 nm).
    c. Argon laser (488nm).
    d. Erbium Laser (1940 nm).

Answers

1. a. Light Amplification by Stimulated Emission of Radiation.
2. a. Theodore Maiman.
3. c. Erbium.
4. a. Nd: YAG Laser.
5. b. Co2 laser.
6. a. Diode laser.
7. d. Helium-Neon laser.
8. a. Argon laser.
9. a. KTP Laser.
10. a. Co2 Laser.
11. b. Diode Laser (633 nm).
12. c. Diode Laser (635 nm).
13. c. Helium-neon Laser (633 nm).
14. a. Helium-neon Laser (633 nm).
15. a. Argon Laser (488 and 515 nm).
16. a. Nd YAG Laser (10600 nm).

Chapter 28

Ozone Therapy and Its Applications in Dentistry

Questions

1. The father of ozone therapy is?
   a. Christian Frederich Schoenbein
   b. Miller
   c. Paatero
   d. William Harvey

2. The first dentist to use ozone therapy in his practice?
   a. E. A. Fisch
   b. Paatero
   c. Miller
   d. Numata

3. The mechanism of action of Ozone includes the following, EXCEPT?
   a. Antimicrobial action
   b. Immunostimulant effect
   c. Hypoxic effect
   d. Biosynthetic effect

4. The mechanism of action of Ozone is by firstly causing damage to the following structure by ozonolysis of double bonds?
   a. Cell membrane
   b. Nucleus
   c. Cytoplasm
   d. DNA

5. The biosynthetic effect of Ozone is caused by the increase in the number of following cell constituents?
   a. Nucleus
   b. Cell membrane and Cytoplasm
   c. Ribosomes and Mitochondria
   d. DNA and RNA

6. Eliminating bacterial pathogens by removing bacterial biofilms from the teeth?
   a. Biofilm Purging
   b. Excision New attachment procedure.
   c. Disclosing agent
   d. Bacteriolysis

7. A compact, easy-to-use tabletop unit with a free flow ozone delivery system utilizes corona discharge. Root canals and periodontal pockets could be easily penetrated?
   a. Ozotop
   b. Nanobubble
   c. Ozonated water
   d. Ozonized olive oil

8. The forms of the ozone-generating system are all the following EXCEPT?
   a. Infrared system
   b. UV System
   c. Cold Plasma system
   d. Corona discharge

9. The dentist uses aqueous Ozone as a powerful disinfectant to control bleeding and cleanse wounds in bone and soft tissues?
   a. Krammer
   b. Miller
   c. Fournier
   d. Slyver

10. Ozone therapy is used to treat?
    a. Osteonecrosis of the jaw.
    b. Haemorrhage.
    c. Hyperthyroidism.
    d. Autoimmune disorders.

Answers

1. a. Christian Frederich Schoenbien.
2. a. E. A. Fisch.
3. c. Hypoxic effect.
4. d. DNA.
5. c. Ribosomes and Mitochondria.
6. a. Biofilm Purging.
7. a. Ozotop.
8. d. Corona discharge.
9. a. Krammer.
10. a. Osteonecrosis of the jaw.

Chapter 29

Nail Changes in Diagnosis of Systemic Disorders

Questions

1. The linear brown-black or red streaks in the basal nail plate called splinter hemorrhages that results from extravasation of blood from the longitudinally oriented vessels of the nail bed are seen in the following disorder?
   a. Infective Endocarditis
   b. Arsenic poisoning
   c. Iron deficiency anemia.
   d. Lichen planus

2. The transverse depressions in the nail plate occur after a stressful event that temporarily interrupts nail formation. They appear first at the cuticle and move distally with nail growth. Beau's lines are more apparent on thumb and great toenails.
   a. Beau's lines.
   b. Mees lines
   c. Leukonychia
   d. Anonychia

3. Spoon-shaped Reverse curvature in the transverse and longitudinal axes giving a concave dorsal aspect to the nail commonly seen in the thumb or greater toe is called?
   a. Koilonychia.
   b. Anonychia
   c. Leukonychia.
   d. Micronychia.

4. A single, transverse, narrow whitish line that runs the width of the nail plate and is seen on multiple nails?
   a. Mee's Lines
   b. Beaus Lines
   c. Lead poisoning.
   d. Bismuth poisoning.

5. The double white transverse lines represent an abnormality of the nail vascular bed and temporarily disappear on squeezing the distal digit. They usually occur on the 2 nd, 3 rd, and 4 th fingernails?
   a. Chronic hypoalbunimia.
   b. Chronic anemia.
   c. Chronic Bulimia.
   d. Chronic Lead poisoning.

6. A form of apparent leukonychia with an average proximal half and a distinctly abnormal brownish distal portion. The distal portion begins proximally where the normal or whitish nail ends and terminates distally where the nail's free end loses its attachment to the hyponychium?
   a. Lindsay's Nails
   b. Mee's Lines
   c. Beau's lines
   d. Koilonychia.

7. The Lindsay's Nails are seen in the following patients?
   a. HIV
   b. Anemia
   c. Cirrhosis
   d. Arsenic poisoning

8. The obliteration of the typical diamond-shaped space formed when the dorsal sides of the distal phalanges of the corresponding right and left digits are opposed?
   a. Schamroth sign.
   b. Leukonychia.
   c. Micronychia.
   d. Reverse halo sign.

9. The following carcinoma can clinically manifest as an increased reddish color of the nail bed due to the production of excess erythropoietin?
   a. Adenocarcinoma of Lung
   b. Renal carcinoma of the Kidney.
   c. Angiosarcoma of Liver
   d. Phaeochromocytoma.

10. The nail changes in hyperthyroidism consist of onycholysis beginning in the fourth or fifth digits?
   a. Plummer's Nail
   b. Terry's Nail
   c. Micronychia.
   d. Leukonychia

11. An extreme form of self-mutilation of digits is?
   a. Obsessive-compulsive disorder.
   b. Manic depressive illness.
   c. Bipolar disorder.
   d. Schizophrenia.

12. Self-mutilation of the digits is seen in the following syndrome?
   a. Lesch -Nyhan syndrome.
   b. Peutz-jeghers synfrome.
   c. Down Syndrome.
   d. Melkerson-rosenthal syndrome.

13. The discontinuance of growth in the nail matrix from the proximal part of the nail and onset of separation of the nail from the nail bed?
   a. onychomadesis.
   b. Anonychia.
   c. Leukonychia.
   d. Koilonychia.

14. What is the rarest adverse effect seen after early valproic acid therapy for epilepsy?
   a. onychomadesis.
   b. Anonychia.
   c. Leukonychia.
   d. Koilonychia.

Answers

1. a. Infective endocarditis.
2. a. Beau's lines.
3. a. Koilonychia.
4. a. Mee's Lines.
5. a. Chronic Hypoalbunimia.
6. a. Lindsay's Nails.
7. c. Cirrhosis.
8. a. Schamroth sign.
9. b. Renal carcinoma of the kidney.
10. a. Plummer's Nail.
11. a. Obsessive-compulsive disorder.
12. a. Lesch Nyhan syndrome.
13. a. Onychomadesis.
14. a. Onychomadesis.

Chapter 30

Clinical Signs in Oral Medicine

Questions

1. The phenomenon in which tiny bleeding points are observed when the white scales are removed in Psoriasis is called?
   a. Auspitz's sign.
   b. Crackers sign.
   c. Crowe's sign.
   d. Bon Bon sign.

2. Tapping of the angle of the jaw cause twitching of the facial muscles called?
   a. Cracker's sign.
   b. Crowe's sign.
   c. Bon Bon sign.
   d. Trousseau's sign.

3. The ability to touch the tip of the nose with the tongue in Ehler Danlos syndrome is?
   a. Gorlin's sign.
   b. Crowe's sign.
   c. Bon Bon sign.
   d. Cracker's sign.

4. The application of lateral pressure in intact skin induces new blisters called?
1. Nikolsky's sign.
2. Crowe's sign.
3. Battle's sign.
4. Auspit'z sign.

5. When pressure is applied to the center of the blister, there will be an extension of the blister near the adjacent intact unblistered skin called?
   a. Asboe Hansen sign.
   b. Crowe's sign.
   c. Auspit'z sign.
   d. Nikolsky's sign.

6. The Axillary characteristic freckling seen in Neurofibromatosis is?
   a. Crowe's sign.
   b. Auspit'z sign.
   c. Nikolsky's sign.
   d. Asboe Hansen sign.

7. The discomfort caused when eating dry foods in Sjogren's syndrome is called?
   a. Cracker's sign.
   b. Crowe's sign.
   c. Coleman's sign.
   d. Chvosteck's sign.

8. The transient bilateral upper lid edema in patients with infectious mononucleosis?
   a. Higoumenaki's sign.
   b. Hutchinson's nose sign.
   c. Hoagland sign.
   d. Bells sign.

9. Crowe's sign occurs in the following disorder?
   a. Neurofibromatosis-Type I.
   b. Pemphigus vegetans.
   c. Bullous Pemphigoid.
   d. Lichen planus.

10. Auspitz sign is seen?
    a. Neurofibromatosis-Type I.
    b. Lichen planus.
    c. Psoriasis.
    d. Pemphigus.

11. The phenomenon called the BonBon sign occur?
    a. Pemphigus.
    b. Lichenplanus.
    c. Tardive dyskinesia.
    d. Type I-Neurofibromatosis.

12. Rosette's sign occurs in the following disorder?
    a. Linear IgA disease.
    b. Lichen planus.
    c. Lupus erythematosus.
    d. Pemphigus.

13. Carpet Tack sign occur in following lesion?
    a. Pemphigus.
    b. Discoid Lupus erythematosus.
    c. Lichen planus.
    d. Leukemia.

14. Comby sign occurs in the following disorder?
    a. Chickenpox.
    b. Varicella.
    c. Measles.
    d. Herpangina.

15. Chvostek sign occurs in the following disorder?
    a. Tetany.
    b. Measles.
    c. Hypercalcemia of Malignancy.
    d. Parkinson's disease.

16. Forchheimer's sign is a feature in?
    a. Measles.
    b. Rubella.
    c. Herpangina.
    d. Herpes zoster.

17. Fournier's sign is seen in?
    a. Staphylococcal scalded skin syndrome.
    b. Congenital syphilis.
    c. Secondary syphilis.
    d. Tertiary Syphilis.

18. Gorlin's sign is a feature of?
    a. Ehlers Danlos syndrome.
    b. Herpangina.
    c. Herpes zoster.
    d. Measles.

19. Mouth mirror sign is due?
    a. Xerostomia.
    b. Ptyalism.
    c. Sialorrhea.
    d. Hypersalivation.

20. Russell's sign is a feature?
    a. Anorexia nervosa.
    b. Xerostomia.
    c. Sialorrhea.
    d. Measles.

Answers

1. a. Auspit'z Sign.
2. d. Trousseau's sign.
3. c. BonBon sign.
4. a. Nikolsy's sign.
5. a. Asboe Hansen Sign.
6. a. Crowe's sign.
7. a. Cracker's sign.
8. c. Hoagland's sign.
9. a. Neurofibromatosis Type I.
10. c. Psoriasis.
11. c. Tardive Dyskinesia.
12. a. Linear IgA Disease.
13. b. Discoid Lupus Erythematosus.
14. c. Measles.
15. a. Tetany.
16. b. Rubella.
17. b. Congenital syphilis.
18. a. Ehler Danlos syndrome.
19. a. Xerostomia.
20. a. Anorexia Nervosa.

Chapter 31

Salivary Diagnostics

Questions

1. The specialized cup used for collecting submandibular saliva?
   a. Lashley cup.
   b. Crimson cup.
   c. Crittenden cup.
   d. Bowen cup.

2. The specialized cup used for the collection of parotid saliva is?
   a. Carlson Crittenden device.
   b. Lashley cup.
   c. Crimson cup.
   d. Ashley cup

3. Palate, Lung, and Nasal epithelium carcinoma-associated Protein 2 (PLUNC2), also known as Parotid secretory protein, was decreased?
   a. Active Periodontitis
   b. Pericoronitis
   c. Gingivitis.
   d. Cellulitis

4. The study of profiling the proteins in saliva throughout disease progression could reveal potential biomarkers indicative of different stages of diseases, which may be helpful in medical diagnostics?
   a. Proteomics
   b. Genomics.
   c. Point of care diagnostics.
   d. Pneumonics

5. An advance, rapid antibody test used as a screening and risk assessment test for HIV?
   a. Oraquick.
   b. Ora risk.
   c. Ora screen.
   d. Perio path.

6. A chairside salivary diagnostic test used to identify the subtypes of Human Papilloma Virus (HPV) is?
   a. Oraquick.
   b. Ora risk.
   c. Ora screen.
   d. Perio-path

7. A salivary diagnostic test based on polymer micropatterned electrodes electric induced deposition that helps identify various systemic diseases?
   a. Oral fluid Nanosensor test (OFNASET)
   b. Ora quick
   c. Salimark.
   d. Vigilant BIO

8. An Antigen-based home test kit approved by Indian council of medical research for COVID-19?
   a. Pathocatch.
   b. OraQuick.
   c. Orasure.
   d. Salimark.

9. The test kit used for detecting oral squamous cell carcinoma by detecting salivary RNA is?
   a. Oraquick.
   b. Orasure.
   c. Peri Rx -Salimark.
   d. Pathocatch.

10. The first Point of care testing device approved for early diagnosis of Nipah virus is?
    a. Orasure.
    b. Peri Rx- Salimark.
    c. Pathocatch.
    d. True-nat.

11. What is the RT-PCR assay-based device for detecting Zika Virus in the saliva?
    a. NucliSENS® easyMAG® system (BioMerieux).
    b. Ora Risk.
    c. True-nat.
    d. Patho-catch.

12. The new component is saliva, which can be used as a biomarker tool to detect oral Squamous cell carcinoma?
    a. Cyfra 21-1 (Tissue Polypeptide antigen).
    b. Matrix metalloproteinases (MMP).
    c. Statherin.
    d. Tumour Necrosis Factor.

Answers

1. a. Lashley Cup.
2. a. Carlson Crittenden device.
3. a. Active Periodontitis.
4. a. Proteomics.
5. a. Ora-quick.
6. b. Ora-risk.
7. a. Oral fluid Nanosensor test (OFNASET)
8. a. Pathocatch.
9. c. Peri-Rx-Salimark.
10. d. True-nat.
11. d. Path-o-catch.
12. a. Cyfra 21-1 (Tissue Polypeptide antigen).

Chapter 32

Immunobiologicals

Questions

1. The monoclonal antibody with promising results in treating squamous cell carcinoma involving the Head and Neck cancers is?
   a. Imatinib.
   b. Bevacuzimab.
   c. Toclizumab.
   d. Efalizumab.

2. The monoclonal antibody used in the treatment of Pemphigus is?
   a. Etanercept.
   b. Bevacuzimab.
   c. Toclizumab.
   d. Imatinib.

3. The monoclonal antibody used in the treatment of Hodgkin's Lymphoma is?
   a. Brentuximab.
   b. Bevacuzimab.
   c. Imatinib.
   d. Daclizumab.

4. The monoclonal antibody directed against CD-33 and used in the treatment of Acute Myeloid Leukemia is?
   a. Gemtuzumab.
   b. Imatinib.
   c. Bevacuzimab.
   d. Daclizumab.

5. The monoclonal antibody used in the treatment of Chronic Lymphocytic Leukemia?
   a. Ofatumumab.
   b. Imatinib.
   c. Tocilizumab.
   d. Bevacuximab.

6. The monoclonal antibody used in the treatment of Asthma?
   a. Mepolizumab.
   b. Imatinib.
   c. Gemtuzumab.
   d. Ranizumab.

7. The monoclonal antibody used in the treatment of Metastatic Malignant Melanoma?
   a. Iplimumab.
   b. Imatinib.
   c. Gemtuzumab.
   d. Toclizumab.

8. The monoclonal antibody used to treat Sjogren's syndrome by targeting B cell-activating factor is?
   a. Belimumab.
   b. Toclizumab.
   c. Imatinib.
   d. Gemtuzumab.

9. The monoclonal antibody used in the treatment of cutaneous T-cell Lymphoma is?
   a. Denileukin Difitox
   b. Denosumab.
   c. Daclizumab.
   d. Tocilizumab.

10. The monoclonal antibody used in treating Systemic Lupus Erythematosus by targeting against Interferon -α?
    a. Rontalizumab.
    b. Daclizumab.
    c. Denosumab.
    d. Tocilizumab.

11. The novel agent used in treating patients with already treated and relapsed or refractory Chronic Lymphocytic Leukemia?
    a. Venetoclax.
    b. Tocilizumab.
    c. Daclizumab.
    d. Denosumab.

12. A novel Bruton's Tyrosine kinase inhibitor used to treat Mantle Cell Lymphoma?
    a. Tocilizumab.
    b. Zanabrutinib.
    c. Daclizumab.
    d. Rontalizumab.

Answers

1. a. Imatinib.
2. a. Etanercept.
3. a. Brentuzimab.
4. a. Gemtuzumab.
5. a. Ofatumumab.
6. a. Mepolizumab.
7. a. Iplimumab.
8. a. Belimumab.
9. a. Denileukin difitox.
10. a. Rontalizumab.
11. a. Venetoclax.
12. b. Zanabrutinib.

Chapter 33

Chairside Investigations and Diagnostic Tests in Oral Medicine

Questions

1. Tooth sloth test is used for diagnosis?
   a. Cracked tooth syndrome.
   b. Pulpitis.
   c. Apical Periodontitis.
   d. Periapical abscess.

2. Pulse oximeter is a device used to measure the following?
   a. Oxygen
   b. oxygen saturation
   c. deoxygenated blood.
   d. Both oxygenated and deoxygenated blood.

3. Hess Test is used?
   a. Neutropenia.
   b. Thrombocytopenia.
   c. Anemia.
   d. Leukemia.

4. Glass test used to detect?
   a. Neutropenia.
   b. Purpura.
   c. Anemia.
   d. Von Willebrand disease.

5. Fremitus test is used to detect?
   a. Trauma from occlusion.
   b. Dental caries.
   c. Gingivitis.
   d. Cervical abrasion.

6. Monospot test or Paul-Bunnell test is?
   a. Glandular fever.
   b. Pel-Ebstein fever.
   c. Tertian fever.
   d. Quartan fever.

7. The person used the first fluorescent disclosing solution?
   a. Skimmer.
   b. Ray Bin.
   c. Skinner.
   d. Lang.

8. The culture medium used to differentiate subspecies of candidiasis is?
   a. Pagano Levine Medium.
   b. Sarbarouds Dextrose Agar Medium.
   c. Chocolate Agar.
   d. Yolk sac culture.

9. What is the chairside test used to identify gustatory sweating in Frey's syndrome?
   a. Starch iodine test.
   b. Tooth sloth test.
   c. Glass test.
   d. Fremitus test.

10. The easiest and fastest way to identify dental plaque is?
    a. Disclosing solution.
    b. Fluorophore.
    c. Haematinic.
    d. Diagnosing solution.

11. Thumb sign occur due to?
    a. Acute epiglottis in children.
    b. Maxillary sinusitis.
    c. Mucormycosis.
    d. Aspergillosis.

12. Black turbinate sign occurs by which fungal infection?
    a. Aspergillosis.
    b. Blastomycosis.
    c. Mucormycosis.
    d. Coccidiomycosis.

13. The chair-side test in which a microscopic glass slide is placed on the surface of a small vascular lesion and whether blanching is observed or not through the glass slide is called?
    a. Spectroscopy.
    b. Microscopy.
    c. Diascopy.
    d. Endoscopy.

14. The test used for diagnosis of contact dermatitis?
    a. Pathergy Test.
    b. Tuberculin Test.
    c. Capillary fragility test.
    d. Patch Test.

15. The test in which an altered tissue response is observed for the formation of Papule or sterile pustule following needle prick?
    a. Patch test.
    b. Pathergy test.
    c. Tuberculin test.
    d. Capillary fragility test.

16. The test used for evaluating the consistency of more minor swellings less than 2 cm in diameter, whether solid or cystic is?
    a. Patch Test.
    b. Paget's Test.
    c. Pathergy test.
    d. Tourniquet Test.

17. Slip sign, in which when the edge of the swelling is palpated with a finger, it slips, characteristically occurs?
    a. Lipoma.
    b. Fibroma.
    c. Neuroma.
    d. Haematoma.

18. The characteristic sign in Haemangioma is?
    a. Reducibility.
    b. Compressibility.
    c. Fixity.
    d. Positivity for Transillumination.

19. Schirmer test is used for evaluation of gland?
    a. Parotid Gland.
    b. Submandibular Gland.
    c. Sublingual Gland.
    d. Lacrimal Gland.

20. The test used to assess caries activity by the principle of salivary micro-organisms producing organic acid from a carbohydrate medium?
    a. Snyder Test.
    b. Salivary Flow test.
    c. Salivary Reductase Test.
    d. Colony Forming Unit Test.

21. The indicator present in Snyder agar, which helps in the formation of green color, when there is a marked caries activity is?
    a. Bromocresol Green.
    b. Dextrose.
    c. Yeast extract.
    d. Casein.

22. The following color change indicates marked caries activity in the salivary reductase test?
    a. Green.
    b. Blue.
    c. Red.
    d. Pink.

Answers

1. a. Cracked Tooth Syndrome.
2. b. Oxygen saturation.
3. b. Thrombocytopenia.
4. b. Purpura.
5. a. Trauma from occlusion.
6. a. Glandular Fever.
7. d. Lang.
8. a. Pagano Levine Medium.
9. a. Starch Iodine test.
10. a. Disclosing solution.
11. a. Acute epiglottis in children.
12. c. Mucormycosis.
13. c. Diascopy.
14. d. Patch test.
15. b. Pathergy test.
16. b. Paget's test.
17. a. Lipoma.
18. b. Compressibility.
19. d. Lacrimal gland.
20. a. Snyder test.
21. a. Bromocresol Green.
22. d. Pink.

Chapter 34

Vitamins and Minerals

Questions

1. The following Vitamin is essential for maintaining epithelial integrity?
    a. Vitamin B12.
    b. Vitamin C.
    c. Vitamin A.
    d. Vitamin E.

2. The Vitamin that acts as a cofactor in the hydroxylation of lysine and proline in collagen formation?
    a. Vitamin A.
    b. Vitamin B.
    c. Vitamin C.
    d. Vitamin E.

3. The Vitamin with a direct action on Parathyroid Hormone?
    a. Vitamin A.
    b. Vitamin B.
    c. Vitamin C.
    d. Vitamin D.

4. The deficiency of Vitamin leads to Scorbutic gingivitis?
    a. Vitamin A.
    b. Vitamin B.
    c. Vitamin C.
    d. Vitamin D.

5. The Vitamin that can cause Enamel Hypoplasia?
    a. Vitamin B.
    b. Vitamin C.
    c. Vitamin D.
    d. Vitamin E.

6. The following mineral is essential for the sensation of Taste?
   a. Zinc.
   b. Selenium.
   c. Manganese.
   d. Phosphorus.

7. The mineral that forms a part of the Hemoglobin molecule in Red Blood cells (Erythrocytes)?
   a. Manganese.
   b. Selenium.
   c. Iron.
   d. Zinc.

8. The mineral that helps in regulating blood glucose levels?
   a. Manganese.
   b. Chromium.
   c. Iron.
   d. Selenium.

9. The mineral found in thyroid hormone?
   a. Zinc.
   b. Iodine.
   c. Selenium.
   d. Manganese.

10. Mineral essential for conduction of nerve transmission?
    a. Zinc.
    b. Selenium.
    c. Chromium.
    d. Calcium.

Answers

1. c. Vitamin A.
2. c. Vitamin C.
3. d. Vitamin D.
4. c. Vitamin C.
5. d. Vitamin E.
6. a. Zinc.
7. c. Iron.
8. b. Chromium.
9. b. Iodine.
10. d. Calcium.

Chapter 35

Antioxidants

Questions

1. The red pigment obtained from the skin of raw tomatoes is?
   a. Lycopene.
   b. Curcumin.
   c. Flavanoids.
   d. Zeaxanthin

2. A yellow-colored pigment that protects the eye from harmful effects of oxidation?
   a. Flavanoids.
   b. Curcumin.
   c. Zeaxanthin.
   d. Lycopene.

3. The major flavonoid that helps to act as a light filter protecting the eye from damage by sunlight?
   a. Lutein.
   b. Lycopene.
   c. Curcumin.
   d. Vitamin C.

4. The natural antioxidant found in Green Tea?
   a. Lutein.
   b. Zeaxanthin.
   c. Epigallocatechin-3-Gallate (EGCG).
   d. Lycopene.

5. The natural antioxidant produced by Curcuma longa (Turmeric)?
   a. Lycopene.
   b. Zeaxanthin.
   c. Lutein.
   d. Curcumin.

6. Which of the following antioxidant has an anti-Ultraviolet action and biosensing and bioimaging applications?
   a. Lignin.
   b. Curcumin.
   c. Lycopene.
   d. Lutein.

7. Which of the following antioxidant helps to promote nerve repair in peripheral nerve injuries?
   a. Lignin.
   b. Curcumin.
   c. Lutein.
   d. Gastrodin.

8. The following is used to reduce toxic aldehyde content in Beer?
   a. White Grape Pomace.
   b. Lycopene.
   c. Lignin.
   d. Lutein.

9. Which of the following is called suicidal antioxidant?
   a. Melatonin.
   b. Lignin.
   c. Gastrodin.
   d. Lutein.

10. Which of the following is a lipophilic antioxidant?
    a. Vitamin E.
    b. Vitamin C.
    c. Vitamin B1.
    d. Vitamin B6.

11. Which of the following is a hydrophilic antioxidant EXCEPT?
    a. Vitamin C.
    b. Bilirubin.
    c. Uric acid.
    d. Ubiquinol.

12. Which of the following antioxidant is an enzyme?
    a. Glutathione peroxidase.
    b. Uric acid.
    c. Albumin.
    d. Thiol.

Answers

1. a. Lycopene.
2. c. Zeaxanthin.
3. a. Lutein.
4. c. Epigallocatechin-3-Gallate (EGCG).
5. d. Curcumin.
6. a. Lignin.
7. d. Gastrodin.
8. a. White Grape Pomace.
9. a. Lycopene.
10. a. Lipophilic antioxidant.
11. d. Ubiquinol.
12. a. Glutathione peroxidase.

Chapter 36

Syndromes of the Head and Neck

Questions

1. The Double Lip is a feature of the following syndrome?
   a. Down Syndrome.
   b. Apert Syndrome.
   c. Crouzon Syndrome.
   d. Vanderwoudes Syndrome.

2. Multiple Odontogenic Keratocysts are a feature of the following syndrome?
   a. Basal cell naevi bifid rib syndrome.
   b. Down Syndrome.
   c. Crouzon syndrome.
   d. Apert syndrome.

3. The syndrome associated with Gingival enlargement?
   a. Rutherford syndrome.
   b. Vanderwoudes syndrome.
   c. Crouzon syndrome.
   d. Apert syndrome.

4. Cleft of the soft palate is associated with the following syndrome?
   a. Velocardiofacial syndrome.
   b. Crouzon syndrome.
   c. Labard Syndrome.
   d. Basal cell naevi bifid rib syndrome.

5. Multiple Pulp stones is a feature of the following syndrome?
   a. Amelogenesis imperfecta.
   b. Marfans syndrome.
   c. Costen syndrome.
   d. Gorlin-Goltz syndrome.

6. Multiple Papillomatous lesions are one manifestation of the following syndrome?
   a. Crouzon syndrome.
   b. Pierre-rhomberg syndrome.
   c. Cowden's syndrome.
   d. Patterson-kelly syndrome.

7. Trotter's syndrome is associated with the following disorder?
   a. Cleft palate.
   b. Carcinoma of the oropharynx.
   c. Carcinoma of the laryngopharynx.
   d. Carcinoma of the nasopharynx.

8. Ramsay hunt syndrome is associated with infection of the following ganglion?
   a. Herpes zoster infection of Geniculate ganglion.
   b. Herpes zoster infection of Trigeminal Ganglion.
   c. Smallpox.
   d. Varicella infection of Trigeminal ganglion.

9. The syndrome associated with Palmar plantar Hyperkeratosis and premature periodontitis?
   a. CREST syndrome.
   b. Ramsay Hunt syndrome.
   c. Papillon-Lefevre syndrome.
   d. Trotter's syndrome.

10. Orogenital ulcerations and chronic ocular inflammation are a feature in?
    a. Adamantiade's syndrome.
    b. Papillon Lefevre syndrome.
    c. Rubenstein Taybi syndrome.
    d. Melkerson Rosenthal syndrome.

11. Nance Horan syndrome is associated with defects?
    a. Enamel.
    b. Dentin.
    c. Pulp.
    d. Root.

12. The increased tendency for a tooth to acquire dental caries occurs in the following syndrome of generalized enamel defects?
    a. Tricho-dental osseous syndrome.
    b. Noonan syndrome.
    c. Papillon -lefevre syndrome.
    d. Melkerson Rosenthal syndrome.

13. Macrocephaly due to hydrocephalus, Macroglossia occurs in the following syndrome?
    a. Tricho-dento osseous syndrome.
    b. Behcet's syndrome.
    c. Melkerson-Rosenthal syndrome.
    d. Maroteaux-Lamy syndrome.

14. The syndrome associated with an inability of infants to make a crying sound due to the deposition of waxy material in laryngeal mucosa and vocal cords is?
    a. Urbach-Wiethe syndrome.
    b. Maroteaux-Lamy syndrome.
    c. Behcet's syndrome.
    d. Rubenstein taybi syndrome.

15. The syndrome is characterized by an underdeveloped mandible, coloboma on the outer portion of eyelid, extra ear tags, or misplaced ears with ossicle defects or absence of external auditory canal leading to conductive hearing loss?
    a. Urbach-Wiethe syndrome.
    b. Francheschetti-Zwahlen-Klein syndrome.
    c. Rubenstein Taybi syndrome.
    d. Apert syndrome.

16. A rare combination of rheumatic mitral stenosis and an atrial septal defect is seen in the following syndrome?
    a. Lutembacher's syndrome.
    b. Reiter syndrome.
    c. Apert syndrome.
    d. Melkerson Rosenthal syndrome.

17. Hemifacial microsomia is a feature of the following syndrome?
    a. Crouzon syndrome.
    b. Goldenhar syndrome.
    c. Pierre robin syndrome.
    d. Marfan syndrome.

18. The syndrome associated with Micrognathia of the mandible is?
    a. Nager syndrome.
    b. Melkerson Rosenthal syndrome.
    c. Proteus syndrome.
    d. Pierre robin syndrome.

19. The syndrome associated with micrognathia, microcephaly, hypotrichosis, underdeveloped nasal cartilage is?
    a. Proteus syndrome.
    b. Melkerson Rosenthal syndrome.
    c. Frey's syndrome.
    d. Hallermann streiff syndrome.

20. Abnormal large sides of the skull, Congenital cataracts, microphthalmia, retinal detachments can occur in the following syndrome?
    a. Francois dyscephaly syndrome.
    b. Melkerson Rosenthal syndrome.
    c. Down Syndrome.
    d. Crouzon syndrome.

21. The syndrome associated with Enamel Hypoplasia, repeated candidiasis, early-onset periodontitis with signs of Liver cirrhosis is?
    a. Melkerson Rosenthal syndrome.
    b. Patterson-Kelly syndrome.
    c. Wilson syndrome.
    d. Cowden syndrome.

22. Gingival enlargement with progressive sensorineural deafness is a feature?
    a. Rutherford syndrome.
    b. Jones syndrome.
    c. Cross syndrome.
    d. Costello syndrome.

23. The syndrome associated with nasal and Perioral Papillomas, Macrostomia, and Gingival enlargement within the first year of life?
    a. Rutherford syndrome.
    b. Cross Syndrome.
    c. Costello syndrome.
    d. Jones syndrome.

24. The syndrome associated with mental retardation, corneal opacity, failure of tooth eruption, Gingival enlargement is?
    a. Cross syndrome.
    b. Cowden syndrome.
    c. Costello syndrome.
    d. Rutherfurd syndrome.

25. The syndrome associated with cherubism, juvenile rheumatoid arthritis, hypertrichosis, Gingival enlargement is?
    a. Cross syndrome.
    b. Ramon syndrome.
    c. Costello syndrome.
    d. Cross syndrome.

26. The syndrome associated with Gingival enlargement, Hyperextensible Metacarpophalangeal joint, Hepatomegaly, and splenomegaly is?
    a. Rutherford syndrome.
    b. Ramon syndrome.
    c. Zimmerman-Laband syndrome.
    d. Costello syndrome.

27. The syndrome associated with Gingival enlargement, midface retraction, ocular hypertelorism, Macroglossia, hydronephrosis due to absence of ureter, Hypospadias?
    a. Schinzel-Giedion syndrome.
    b. Zimmerman- Laband syndrome.
    c. Ramon syndrome.
    d. Rutherford syndrome.
28. Bilateral sternoclavicular joint edema, recurrent multifocal osteomyelitis, Palmoplantar Pustulosis is a feature of the following syndrome?
    a. SAPHO Syndrome.
    b. Costello syndrome.
    c. Cross syndrome.
    d. Costen syndrome.

29. The syndrome associated with otalgia due to decreased vertical dimension in edentulous Patients?
    a. Costello syndrome.
    b. Cross syndrome.
    c. Cowden syndrome.
    d. Costen syndrome.

30. The syndrome associated with renal failure due to crushing injury to skeletal muscle?
    a. By-Waters syndrome.
    b. Costen syndrome.
    c. Ramon syndrome.
    d. Cross syndrome.

31. The syndrome associated with Taurodontism, enamel hypoplasia, cryptorchidism (undescended testes)?
    a. Rubenstein-Taybi syndrome.
    b. Klinefelter syndrome.
    c. Marfan syndrome.
    d. Melkerson Rosenthal syndrome.

32. The syndrome associated with Talon cusp, short stature, hearing loss, low intellectual ability, down slanted palpebral fissures, low hanging columella?
    a. Marfan syndrome.
    b. Melkerson Rosenthal syndrome.
    c. Klinefelter syndrome.
    d. Rubenstein Taybi syndrome.

33. The syndrome associated with adrenal gland failure caused by bleeding and hemorrhage into the adrenal glands due to bacterial infections like Cytomegalovirus and Neisseria meningitis (Meningococcus)?
    a. Melkerson Rosenthal syndrome.
    b. Klinefelter syndrome.
    c. Waterhouse -Friderichsen syndrome.
    d. Rubenstein-Taybi syndrome.

34. The syndrome associated with Amelogenesis imperfecta?
    a. Tricho dento-osseous syndrome.
    b. Klinefelter syndrome.
    c. Rubenstein-Taybi syndrome.
    d. Melkeron Rosenthal syndrome.

35. The syndrome associated with Amelogenesis imperfecta, infantile-onset epilepsy, intellectual disability with or without dementia?
    a. Rubenstein taybi syndrome.
    b. Marfan syndrome.
    c. Kohlschutter-Tonz syndrome.
    d. Melkerson Rosenthal syndrome.

36. The syndrome of cleft palate, vertical maxillary excess, malar flattening, narrow palpebral fissure, mandibular retrusion, small ears?
    a. Velocardiofacial syndrome.
    b. Melkerson-rosenthal syndrome.
    c. Marfan syndrome.
    d. Rubenstein-Taybi syndrome.

Answers

1. d. Vanderwoudes syndrome.
2. a. Basal cell Naevi Bifid rib syndrome.
3. a. Rutherford syndrome.
4. a. Velocardiofacial syndrome.
5. b. Marfan's syndrome.
6. c. Cowden's syndrome.
7. d. Carcinoma of Nasopharynx.
8. a. Herpes Zoster infection of the Geniculate Ganglion.
9. c. Papillon- Levefre syndrome.
10. a. Adamantiade's syndrome.
11. a. Enamel.
12. a. Tricho-dento osseous syndrome.
13. d. Marteaoux-Lamy syndrome.
14. a. Urbach-wiethe syndrome.
15. b. Francheschetti-Zwahlen-Klein syndrome.
16. a. Lutembacher's syndrome.
17. a. Crouzon syndrome.
18. a. Nager syndrome.
19. a. Proteus syndrome.
20. d. Crouzon syndrome.
21. a. Melkerson Rosenthal syndrome.
22. b. Jones syndrome.
23. c. Costello syndrome.
24. d. Rutherford syndrome.
25. d. Cross syndrome.
26. b. Ramon syndrome.
27. a. Shinzel -Giedion syndrome.
28. a. Sapho syndrome.
29. d. Costen syndrome.
30. a. By-Waters syndrome.
31. b. Klinefelter syndrome.
32. d. Rubenstein Taybi syndrome.
33. c. Waterhouse -Friderichsen syndrome.
34. a. Tricho dento-osseous syndrome.
35. c. Kohlschutter-Tonz syndrome.
36. a. Velocardiofacial syndrome.

Chapter 37

Pharmacotherapies in Dentistry

Questions

1. The drug of choice for Postherpetic Neuralgia is?
   a. Gabapentin.
   b. Ketorolac.
   c. Ibuprofen.
   d. Aceclofenac.

2. The drug of choice for Cytomegalovirus retinitis?
   a. Foscarnet.
   b. Gabapentin.
   c. Acyclovir.
   d. Zidovudine.

3. The dose of Acyclovir for the treatment of Herpes zoster in adults?
   a. 800 mg five times daily.
   b. 200 mg five times daily.
   c. 400 mg five times daily.
   d. 100 mg five times daily.

4. The antifungal used as salvage therapy to treat Mucormycosis?
   a. Posaconazole.
   b. Amphotericin-B.
   c. Fluconazole.
   d. Ketoconazole.

5. The antibiotic of choice for anaerobic infections like abscesses?
   a. Metronidazole.
   b. Amoxicillin.
   c. Ketoconazole.
   d. Itraconazole.

6. Which of the following antibiotic has better penetration in bone?
   a. Clindamycin.
   b. Erythromycin.
   c. Soframycin.
   d. Amoxicillin.

7. The antibiotic-associated with red man syndrome is?
   a. Vancomycin.
   b. Ketoconazole.
   c. Acyclovir.
   d. Erythromycin.

8. The Nonsteroidal anti-inflammatory drug used after an attack of Myocardial infarction post angioplasty procedure?
   a. Aspirin.
   b. Ibuprofen.
   c. Ketorolac.
   d. Aceclofenac.

9. The analgesic contraindicated in young patients below four years of age?
   a. Aspirin.
   b. Ibuprofen.
   c. Ketorolac.
   d. Aceclofenac.

10. The Nonsteroidal anti-inflammatory drug can cause Reyes syndrome, a form of acute encephalitis caused in children associated with fever, skin rash?
    a. Ketorolac.
    b. Ibuprofen.
    c. Aceclofenac.
    d. Aspirin.

11. Which of the topical local anesthetic gel contains Lidocaine in the following concentration?
    a. 5%
    b. 15%
    c. 2%
    d. 20%

12. The spray form of Lidocaine contains the following concentration?
    a. 2%
    b. 3%
    c. 15%
    d. 40%

13. The drug of choice for Burning Mouth Syndrome is?
    a. Clonazepam Lozenges.
    b. Benzotriazole Lozenges.
    c. Nystatin Lozenges.
    d. Nystatin pastilles.

14. The drug of choice in treating trigeminal neuralgia, the advantage of once-daily dosing is needed because of longer shelf life is?
    a. Eslicarbamazepine.
    b. Carbamazepine.
    c. Oxycarbamazepine.
    d. Voriconazole.

15. What is the drug of choice for causing dry oral, nasal, and pharyngeal secretions before and during General anesthesia?
    a. Glycopyrollate.
    b. Pilocarpine.
    c. Cevimeline.
    d. Amifostine.

16. What is the drug of choice for reducing Xerostomia in patients undergoing head and neck radiotherapy for cancer?
    a. Amifostine.
    b. Pilocarpine.
    c. Cevimeline.
    d. Glycopyrollate.

17. The sialogogue contraindicated in patients affected?
    a. Diabetes.
    b. Asthma.
    c. Epilepsy.
    d. Hypertension.

18. What is the recommended dose of sialogogue Pilocarpine for treating Xerostomia due to salivary hypofunction?
    a. 5 mg thrice daily for 12 weeks.
    b. 2mg thrice daily for 12 weeks.
    c. 10 mg thrice daily for 12 weeks.
    d. 15 mg thrice daily for 12 weeks.

19. The recommended dose of cevimeline hydrochloride to treat salivary hypofunction is?
    a. 10 mg Thrice daily.
    b. 20 mg Twice daily.
    c. 30 mg Thrice daily.
    d. 40 mg Twice daily.

20. The antibiotic prophylaxis is mandatory for the following?
    a. Any repaired congenital heart defect by surgery or cardiac catheter intervention during the first six months after the Procedure.
    b. Congenital heart defect treated by cardiac catheter intervention after six months of the Procedure.
    c. Any repaired congenital heart defect by surgery or cardiac catheter intervention during the first three months after the Procedure.
    d. Congenital heart defect treated by cardiac catheter intervention after three months of the Procedure.

21. The drug of choice to treat severe aphthous stomatitis is?
    a. 0.05% Beclomethasone.
    b. 0.1% isotretinoin gel.
    c. 1% Lidocaine gel.
    d. 2.5% Beclomethasone.

22. The significant adverse effect of long-term use of Topical corticosteroids is?
    a. Oral Candidiasis.
    b. Oral Hairy Leukoplakia.
    c. Oral Lichen Planus.
    d. Discoid Lupus Erythematosus.

23. The drug of choice for patients allergic to Penicillin group of drugs is?
    a. Clindamycin 600 mg 1 hour before the Procedure.
    b. Ampicillin 500 mg 1 hour before the Procedure.
    c. Amoxicillin 500 mg 1 hour before the Procedure.
    d. Piperacillin 200 mg 1 hour before the Procedure.

24. The metabolite of chlorzoxazone is implicated in the functioning of kidneys. Hence must it be avoided in patients with renal impairment?
    a. 6-hydroxychlorzoxazone.
    b. 5-hydroxychlorzoxazone.
    c. 4-hydroxychlorzoxazone.
    d. 3-hydroxychlorzoxazone.

25. The muscle relaxant that increases the anti-inflammatory effect of Ketorolac is?
    a. Chlorzoxazone.
    b. Tizanidine.
    c. Metaxalone.
    d. Cyclobenzaprine.

26. The muscle relaxant that can cause arrhythmias and hence contraindicate in patients with cardiac arrhythmias?
    a. Cyclobenzaprine.
    b. Metaxalone.
    c. Tizanidine.
    d. Chlorzoxazone.

27. The newer drug of choice with a longer half-life of 23 hours and hence indicated as once-daily dosage in Trigeminal Neuralgia is?
    a. Carbamazepine.
    b. Oxycarbamazepine.
    c. Eslicarbazepine.
    d. Tetracarbazepine.

28. Lignocaine injection is contraindicated in the following region?
    a. Tip of toes.
    b. Buccal Mucosa.
    c. Lip.
    d. Labial Mucosa.

29. The following drug used to treat iron overload in patients with renal failure for renal dialysis can induce the formation of Mucormycosis?
    a. Desferrioxamine.
    b. Ferrous ascorbate.
    c. Ferrous Fumarate.
    d. Ferric hydroxide.

Answers

1. a. Gabapentin.
2. b. Foscarnet.
3. c. 800 mg five times daily.
4. a. Posoconazole.
5. a. Metronidazole.
6. a. Clindamycin.
7. a. Red man syndrome.
8. a. Aspirin.
9. c. Ketorolac.
10. d. Aspirin.
11. c. 2%.
12. c. 15%.
13. a. Clonazepam lozenges.
14. a. Eslicarbamazepine.
15. a. Glycopyrollate.
16. a. Amifostine.
17. b. Asthma.
18. a. 5mg thrice daily for 12 weeks.
19. c. 30 mg thrice daily.
20. a. Any repaired congenital heart defect by surgery or cardiac catheter intervention during the first six months after the Procedure.
21. a. 0.05% Beclomethasone.
22. a. Oral candidiasis.
23. a. clindamycin 600 mg 1 hour before the Procedure.
24. a. 6-hydroxychlorzoxazone.
25. d. Cyclobenzaprine.
26. a. Cyclobenzaprine.
27. c. Eslicarbazepine.
28. a. Tip of the toes.
29. a. Desferrioxamine.

Chapter 38

Occupational Disorders of the Oral Cavity

Questions

1. The disorder seen among sugar refineries, Bakery and Confectionaries, candy makers is?
   a. Dental caries.
   b. Periodontitis.
   c. Gingivitis.
   d. Abscess.

2. The teeth disorder is commonly seen among cement and sand workers, stone grinders, stone cutters, and miners in the Graphite industry?
   a. Cervical abrasion.
   b. Attrition.
   c. Abfraction.
   d. Erosion.

3. The teeth disorder commonly occurs among musicians, who use brass instruments that impinge on the front teeth?
   a. Yellow stain.
   b. Green stain.
   c. Black stain.
   d. Blue stain.

4. Which of the following can occur in people working in Match Factories?
   a. Habsburg jaw.
   b. Phossy jaw.
   c. Lumpy Jaw.
   d. Pharyngeal Jaw.

5. The most common disorder seen among People working in Aluminium Plants is?
   a. Dental Fluorosis.
   b. Periodontitis.
   c. Dental caries.
   d. Gingivitis.

6. The most common disorder seen among manufacturers of Thermometers and Barometers?
   a. Dental caries.
   b. Cervical abrasion.
   c. Attrition.
   d. Gingivitis.

7. The use of Manganese in dyeing, printing, and bleaching industries lead?
   a. Yellow stain.
   b. Black stain.
   c. Green stain.
   d. Blue stain.

8. The oral cavity disorder caused by the exposure of chromic acid and chromates among workers in the chromium electroplating industry?
   a. Blue pigmentation of oral mucosa.
   b. Yellow pigmentation of the oral mucosa.
   c. Greyish pigmentation of the oral mucosa.
   d. Green pigmentation of the oral mucosa.

9. The most common disorder seen in teeth among cryolite workers, used in metallurgy?
   a. Mottling of teeth.
   b. Dental caries.
   c. Dental Attrition.
   d. Cervical Abrasion.

10. The term "Phossy Jaw" refers to bone affected?
    a. Bone Necrosis.
    b. Retarded Growth of Jaw.
    c. Prognathic Jaws.
    d. Retrognathic Jaws.

Answers

1. a. Dental caries.
2. a. Cervical abrasion.
3. b. Green stain.
4. b. Phossy jaw.
5. a. Dental Fluorosis.
6. d. Gingivitis.
7. b. Black stain.
8. b. Yellow Pigmentation of the oral mucosa.
9. a. Mottling of teeth.
10. a. Bone Necrosis.

Part 2. Radiology

Chapter 39

History of Radiology

Questions

1. The person discovered x-rays?
   a. Alexander Flemming.
   b. Wilhelm Conrad Roentgen.
   c. Marx.
   d. Black. G. V.

2. Who is called the father of dental radiology?
   a. Wilhelm Conrad roentgen.
   b. Louis Pasteur.
   c. G. V. Black.

3. The first dental radiograph was made by?
   a. Edmund Kells.
   b. Wilhelm Conrad roentgen.
   c. Louis Pasteur.
   d. Otto walkhoff.

4. Who is called the father of radiation Protection?
   a. William Herbert Rollins.
   b. Edmund Kells.
   c. Otto Walkhoff.
   d. Louis Pasteur.

5. Who is credited with the first practical use of radiology in dentistry?
   a. Edmund Kells.
   b. Lars Leskell.
   c. Otto Walkhoff.
   d. James Chadwick.

6. The "Long-distance Technique" to prevent a shadow of the Malar (Zygomatic) bone over the apices of the images of the Maxillary Molars in the Maxillary Molar region was described by the person; named?
   a. Otto Walkhoff.
   b. Mc Cormack.
   c. Godfrey Hounsfield.
   d. Numata.

7. The Long cone or Paralleling angle Technique was invented?
   a. Gordon Fitzgerald.
   b. Numata.
   c. Godfrey Hounsfield.
   d. Otto Walkhoff.

8. The first machine-made film Packets in dentistry?
   a. Becks.
   b. Eastman Kodak company.
   c. Hounsfield.
   d. Felix Bloch.

9. The Bitewing technique was introduced?
   a. Fitzgerald.
   b. Hounsfield.
   c. Raper. H. R.
   d. Felix Bloch.

10. The inventor of the orthopantomographic machine is?
    a. Numata and Paatero.
    b. Godfrey Hounsfield.
    c. Felix Bloch and Purcell.
    d. Otto Walkhoff.

11. The Electron Beam Computed Tomography was introduced?
    a. Andrew Castagnini.
    b. Numata.
    c. Otto Walkoff.
    d. Hounsfield.

12. Who discovered intensifying screens?
    a. Max Levy.
    b. Numata.
    c. Hounsfield.
    d. Felix Bloch.

13. Who discovered moving Grids?
    a. Max Levy.
    b. Andrew Castagnini.
    c. Numata.
    d. Gustav Bucky.

14. The first radiographic images of the skull?
    a. William J Morton.
    b. Otto Walkhoff.
    c. Numata.
    d. Wilhem Conrad Roentgen

15. Who is called the father of Dental Radiology?
    a. Charles Edmund Kells
    b. Otto Walkhoff.
    c. Wilhem Conrad Roentgen.
    d. Numata.

Answers

1. b. Wilhelm Conrad Roentgen.
2. d. Edmund Kells.
3. d. Otto Walkhoff.
4. a. William Herbert Rollins.
5. a. Edmund Kells.
6. b. Mc Cormack.
7. a. Gordon Fitzgerald.
8. b. Eastman Kodak Company.
9. c. Raper. H. R.
10. a. Numata and Paatero.
11. a. Andrew Castagnini.
12. a. Max Lewy.
13. d. Gustav Bucky.
14. a. William J Morton.
15. a. Charles Edmund Kells.

Chapter 40

Discoveries in Radiology

Questions

1. Who discovered electrons?
   a. Alexander Fleming.
   b. Roentgen.
   c. Chadwick.
   d. Joseph John Thompson.

2. Who discovered Protons?
   a. Roentgen.
   b. Rutherford.
   c. Millikan.
   d. J. J. Thompson.

3. Who discovered Neutrons?
   a. Roentgen.
   b. Millikan.
   c. James Chadwick.
   d. J. J. Thompson.

4. Who discovered alpha particles?
   a. James Chadwick.
   b. Ernest Rutherford.
   c. Millikan.
   d. Gustav ising.

5. Who discovered beta particles?
   a. Ernest Rutherford.
   b. Millikan.
   c. Gustav ising.
   d. Roentgen.

6. Who discovered Gamma rays?
   a. Ernest Rutherford.
   b. Roentgen.
   c. Paul Villard.
   d. Gustav ising.

7. Who discovered cyclotron?
   a. Ernest Rutherford.
   b. Ernest. O. Lawrence.
   c. Paul Villard.
   d. Gustav ising.

8. Who discovered the synchrotron?
   a. Ernest. o. Lawrence.
   b. Paul Villard.
   c. Vladimir Veksler.
   d. Roentgen.

9. Who introduced the term "Panoramic radiography"?
   a. Y. V. Paatero and H. Numata.
   b. Ernest. O. Lawrence.
   c. Vladimir Veksler.
   d. Roentgen.

10. Who discovered the Gamma knife?
    a. Lars Leksell.
    b. Vladimir Veksler.
    c. Paatero.
    d. Roentgen.

11. Who discovered the Gamma camera or scintillation camera?
    a. Lars Leksell.
    b. Vladimir Veksler.
    c. Paatero.
    d. Hal O. Anger.

12. Who discovered Fluoroscopy?
    a. Thomas Edison.
    b. Paatero.
    c. Hal. O. Anger.
    d. Roentgen.

13. Who discovered the Positron Emission Tomography scanner?
    a. Thomas Edison and Michael. E. Phelps.
    b. Hal. O. Anger.
    c. Edward. J. Hoffman.
    d. Numata.

14. Who developed the first dedicated head SPECT?
    a. Ronald Jaszczak.
    b. Paatero.
    c. Edward. J. Hoffman.
    d. Roentgen.

15. Who discovered Helium?
    a. Jules Janssen.
    b. Paatero.
    c. Thomas Edison.
    d. Roentgen.

16. Who discovered the Periodic table in which their atomic number and chemical characteristics arrange the elements?
    a. Dmitri Mendeleev.
    b. Thomas Edison.
    c. Roentgen.
    d. Hal. O. Anger.

17. Who is the father of medical ultrasound?
    a. John. J Wild.
    b. Thomas Edison.
    c. Hal. O. Anger.
    d. Dmitri Mendeleev.

18. Who invented SPECT (Single Photon Emission Computed Tomography)?
    a. Hal. O. Anger.
    b. Paatero.
    c. John Keyes.
    d. Roentgen.

Answers

1. d. Joseph John Thompson.
2. b. Rutherford.
3. c. James Chadwick.
4. b. Ernest Rutherford.
5. a. Ernest Rutherford.
6. c. Paul Villard.
7. b. Ernest. O. Lawrence.
8. c. Vladimir Veksler.
9. a. Y. V. Paatero and H. Numata.
10. a. Lars Leksell.
11. d. Hal. O. Anger.
12. a. Thomas Edison.
13. a. Thomas Edison and Michael E. Phelps.
14. a. Ronald Jaszczak.
15. a. Jules Jannsen.
16. a. Dimitri Mendelev.
17. a. John. J. Wild.
18. c. John Keyes.

Chapter 41

Radiation Physics

Questions

1. The fundamental unit of any particular element cannot be subdivided by any special high energy techniques or ordinary chemical methods?
   a. Element.
   b. Atom.
   c. Nucleus.
   d. Molecule.

2. A sufficiently stable electrically neutral group of at least two atoms in a definite arrangement held together by solid chemical bonds is called?
   a. Atom.
   b. Molecule.
   c. Nucleus.
   d. Orbit.

3. Anything that has mass and occupies space is called?
   a. Matter.
   b. Atom.
   c. Molecule.
   d. Free radical.

4. All stable matter in the universe comprises?
   a. Up Quarks.
   b. Down Quarks.
   c. Electrons.
   d. All the above.

5. Which matter forms the neutrons and Protons in the atomic nuclei?
   a. Up Quarks.
   b. Down Quarks.
   c. Both Up Quarks and Down Quarks.
   d. None of the above.

6. Which of the following model describes the arrangement of electrons in an atom?
    a. Quantum Mechanical Model.
    b. Standard Model.
    c. Bohr Model.
    d. Atomic model.

7. Which force carrier particle mediates strong nuclear force that binds the Protons and Neutrons in the atom's Nuclei?
    a. Photon.
    b. W Bason.
    c. Z Bason.
    d. Gluon.

8. The force carrier particle associated with the decay of beta rays?
    a. W Bason.
    b. Z Bason.
    c. Gluon.
    d. Photon.

9. The force carrier particle associated with Neutrino scatter?
    a. W Bason.
    b. Z Bason.
    c. Photon.
    d. Glucon.

10. Which of the following determines the Atomic number?
    a. Protons.
    b. Electrons.
    c. Neutrons.
    d. Photons.

11. The Atomic Mass refers to the total of the following particles?
    a. Protons and Electrons.
    b. Neutrons and Electrons.
    c. Protons and Neutrons.
    d. Electrons and Neutrons.

12. The change in these affects the stability of the element?
    a. Protons.
    b. Electrons.
    c. Photons.
    d. Neutrons.

13. The probability location of the electrons in the three-dimensional volumes in space at any instant in time is called?
    a. Orbitals.
    b. Mass.
    c. Element.
    d. Atom.

14. The first orbital is designated by the letter?
    a. s
    b. P
    c. d
    d. f
    e. g

15. The shape of the s-orbital is?
    a. Elliptical.
    b. Circular.
    c. Ellipsoidal.
    d. Spherical.

16. The p-orbital is?
    a. Uni-lobed.
    b. Bi-lobed.
    c. Tri-lobed.
    d. Quadri-lobed.

17. The d-type orbitals are?
    a. Uni-lobed with a ring.
    b. Bi-lobed with a ring.
    c. Tri-lobed with a ring.
    d. Quadri-lobed with a ring.

18. An atom is said to be electrically neutral if?
    a. The number of Protons is equal to the number of Neutrons.
    b. The number of electrons is equal to the number of neutrons.
    c. The number of electrons is equal to the number of Protons.
    d. The number of Photons is equal to the number of Protons.

19. A known atom that has no more than the following orbitals?
    a. Six orbitals.
    b. Seven orbitals.
    c. Eight orbitals.
    d. Nine orbitals.

20. The following refers to the rate of energy loss from a particle, as it moves along the track through tissue is called?
    a. Linear Energy Transfer.
    b. Half Value Layer.
    c. Radioactivity.
    d. Ionization.

21. The elementary charge of an alpha particle is?
    a. +1
    b. +2
    c. -1
    d. -2

22. The elementary charge of an electron is?
    a. -1
    b. -2
    c. +1
    d. +2

23. The theory that considers electromagnetic radiation as small discrete bundles of energy?
    a. Quantum theory.
    b. Wave theory.
    c. Standard model.
    d. Bohr model.

24. The energy acquired by one electron accelerates through a potential volt difference?
    a. Electron volt (eV)
    b. Milli amperage (m A)
    c. Kilo voltage peak (kvp)
    d. Sievert(sv)

25. The theory is more helpful in considering radiation in bulk in experiments dealing with refraction, reflection, diffraction, interference, polarization?
    a. Wave theory.
    b. Quantum theory.
    c. Standard model.
    d. Bohr model.

26. The cathode in the dental x-ray tube comprises the following filament?
    a. Copper.
    b. Molybdenum.
    c. Tungsten.
    d. Silver.

27. The diameter and length of the tungsten wire used in the cathode are?
    a. 2mm; 1 cm.
    b. 1mm; 1cm.
    c. 3 mm, 2 cm.
    d. 4mm, 3 cm.

28. The electron beam is focused electrostatically is directed in a small rectangular area on the anode?
    a. Cathode.
    b. Focusing cup.
    c. Anode.
    d. Copper stem.

29. The shape of the Focusing cup in the x-ray tube is?
    a. Parabolic concave.
    b. Parabolic convex.
    c. Elliptical.
    d. Circular.

30. The primary purpose of vacuum inside the x-ray tube is?
    a. Oxidation.
    b. Reduction.
    c. Ionization.
    d. Adsorption.

31. The atomic number of Tungsten filament is?
    a. 71
    b. 72
    c. 73
    d. 74

32. The melting point of Tungsten filament is?
    a. 3122-degree celcius.
    b. 3222-degree celcius.
    c. 3322-degree celcius.
    d. 3422-degree celcius.

33. The thermal conductivity of Tungsten is?
    a. 176 W m-1 k-1.
    b. 177 W m-1 k-1.
    c. 178 W m-1k-1.
    d. 179 W m-1 k-1.

34. The area on the target anode, where electrons from the cathode are directed by focusing cup to falls on the particular site on the anode is called?
    a. Hot spot.
    b. cold spot.
    c. Focal spot.
    d. Hot nodule.

35. The apparent size of the focal spot seen from the position perpendicular to the direction of an electron beam is called?
    a. Actual Focal spot.
    b. Effective focal spot.
    c. Focal trough.
    d. Focal zone.

36. The target anode is inclined at these degrees to the central ray of the x-ray beam?
    a. 10°
    b. 20°
    c. 5°
    d. 15°

37. The effective focal spot in the x-ray tube is?
    a. 1 x 3 mm.
    b. 2 x 1 mm.
    c. 1 x 2 mm.
    d. 2 x 3 mm.

38. The actual Focal spot in the x-ray tube is?
    a. 1 x 1mm.
    b. 1 x 2 mm.
    c. 1 x 3 mm.
    d. 1 x 4 mm.

39. In Rotating anodes, the focal spot is called?
    a. Focal trough.
    b. Focal track.
    c. Actual focal trough.
    d. Effective focal trough.

40. The tube current for operating rotating anodes is?
    a. 100-500 milliamperes.
    b. 200-500 milliamperes.
    c. 300-500 milliamperes.
    d. 400-500 milliamperes.

41. The rotating anodes are used?
    a. Intraoral periapical radiograph units.
    b. Occlusal radiography.
    c. Cone beam units.
    d. Bitewing radiography.

42. The stator coils drive the Rotor in a rotating anode?
    a. 2000 revolutions per minute.
    b. 3000 revolutions per minute.
    c. 4000 revolutions per minute.
    d. 5000 revolutions per minute.

43. What is the kilovoltage Peak of intraoral, panoramic, and cephalometric machines?
    a. 60 and 90 KVp.
    b. 50 and 80 KVp.
    c. 40 and 80 KVp.
    d. 50 and 90 KVp.

44. The cone-beam computed tomographic machines operate at the following kilo-voltage peak?
    a. 60- 90 KVp.
    b. 70-90 KVp.
    c. 90-120 KVp.
    d. 90-110 KVp.

45. The power supply circuitry in which the alternating high voltage is applied directly across the x-ray tube limits the x-ray production to half the Alternating current cycle is called?
    a. Self-rectified
    b. Full-wave rectified.
    c. Non-self-rectified.
    d. Autorectified.

46. When the x-ray tube is powered with 60 cycle AC, the pulses of x-rays generated each second with a duration of following seconds?
    a. 50; 1/120 second.
    b. 60; 1/120 second.
    c. 70; 1/120 second.
    d. 80; 1/120 second.

47. The images produced by full-wave rectified dental x-ray machines, compared to half-wave rectified devices, have these advantages?
    a. Long contrast scale, Lower dose to the patient.
    b. Smaller contrast scale, high dose to the patient.
    c. Minimal contrast, low dose to the patient.
    d. Minimal contrast, High scale to patient.

48. The formula calculates the exposure time in an x-ray tube?
    a. The number of Pulses / Frequency of Power source.
    b. Frequency of Power source / Number of Pulses.
    c. The number of Pulses x Frequency of Power source.
    d. The number of Pulses + Frequency of Power source.

49. Setting 30 pulses of radiation equals?
    a. 0.3-second exposure.
    b. 0.4-second exposure.
    c. 0.5-second exposure.
    d. 0.6-second exposure.

50. The heat produced near the dental x-ray tube's anode is expressed in the following unit?
    a. Hertz.
    b. Heat units.
    c. Kerma.
    d. Adsorbed dose.

51. Is the heat storage capacity of anodes in dental diagnostic x-ray tubes approximate?
    a. 10 KHU.
    b. 20 KHU.
    c. 30 KHU.
    d. 40 KHU.

52. The longest exposure time, the tube can be energized for a range of Voltages (kVp) and Tube current (mA) values without risk of damage to the target from overheating?
    a. Tube rating.
    b. Duty cycle.
    c. Exposure time.
    d. Kerma.

53. The following parameter describes the frequency with which successive exposures can be made without overheating the anode?
    a. Tube rating.
    b. Duty cycle.
    c. Exposure time.
    d. Equivalent dose.

54. A typical Duty cycle in an x-ray tube is?
    a. 1:40
    b. 1:50
    c. 1:60
    d. 1:70

55. The Heat units in the x-ray tube are given by formula?
    a. HU = Kvp x mA x seconds.
    b. HU = kvp x HUX HU
    c. HU= mA X seconds.
    d. HU = Kvp x seconds

56. The element does not have neutral neutrons?
    a. Oxygen.
    b. Hydrogen.
    c. Carbon dioxide.
    d. Nitrogen.

57. The emission and propagation of energy through space or a substance in waves or particles?
    a. Radiation.
    b. Atom.
    c. Element.
    d. Radioactivity.

58. The process by which certain unstable atoms or elements undergo spontaneous disintegration or decay to attain a more balanced nuclear state is called?
    a. Radiation.
    b. Radioactivity.
    c. Radioresponsiveness.
    d. Radiocurability.

59. The electromagnetic waves used in high altitude transmission satellites are called?
    a. Grenz rays.
    b. Hertzian waves.
    c. Radio waves.
    d. Communication waves.

60. The filter in the dental x-ray tube comprises the following element?
    a. Copper.
    b. Tungsten.
    c. Molybdenum.
    d. Aluminum.

61. The inherent filter in the x-ray tube is produced by the following EXCEPT?
    a. The glass wall of an x-ray tube.
    b. Insulating oil.
    c. Barrier material that prevents oil from escaping.
    d. Copper.

62. The added filtration comprises disks made of the following material in a dental x-ray tube?
    a. Copper.
    b. Tungsten.
    c. Molybdenum.
    d. Aluminum.

63. The Metallic barrier used to restrict the size of the x-ray beam and the volume of tissue irradiated is?
    a. Collimator.
    b. Filter.
    c. Focal trough.
    d. Focal spot.

64. The size of the dental x-ray beam is usually collimated to the following diameter on the patient's face?
    a. 5 cm.
    b. 6 cm.
    c. 7 cm.
    d. 8 cm.

65. When x-rays interact with matter, the x-ray photons ionize absorber atoms, convert their energy into the ejected electron's kinetic energy, and cease to exist. This interaction of x-ray is called?
    a. Absorption interactions.
    b. Scattering interactions.
    c. Bremmstraulaug radiation.
    d. Chemical interaction.

66. The interactions of the x-ray photons, in which the photons interact with absorber atoms but then move off in another direction, are called?
    a. Scattering interactions.
    b. Absorption interactions.
    c. Bremmstraulaug radiation.
    d. Mechanical interaction.

67. When the x-ray beam is directed at a patient, the X-ray beam's percentage of the x-ray beam gets absorbed and passes through the patient is?
    a. 90% absorbed, 10% pass-through.
    b. 50% absorbed, 50% pass-through.
    c. 10% absorbed, 90 % Pass-through.
    d. 60% absorbed, 40 % Pass-through.

68. Photons in the x-ray beam primarily interact with the patient resulting from the following?
    a. Coherent scattering.
    b. Photoelectric absorption.
    c. Compton scattering.
    d. Do not interact.

69. The following x-ray interaction produces the least number of interactions of the x-ray beam on a patient?
    a. Coherent scattering.
    b. Compton scattering.
    c. Photoelectric absorption.
    d. No interactions.

70. The Primary contributor to image, hence this is more critical in diagnostic imaging is?
    a. Photoelectric absorption.
    b. Compton scattering.
    c. Coherent scattering.
    d. No interactions.

71. The Photoelectric absorption depends on the frequency of photoelectric interaction varying directly with the following power of the atomic number of the absorber?
    a. First.
    b. Second.
    c. Third.
    d. Fourth.

72. The Photoelectric absorption in bone is approximately greater than soft tissue?
    a. times
    b. 6.5 times
    c. 7.5 times
    d. 8.5 times

73. The Penetrating quality of the x-ray beam is determined by the following?
    a. Half value layers.
    b. Collimator thickness.
    c. Filter thickness.
    d. Lead thickness.

Answers

1. b. Atom.
2. b. Molecule.
3. a. Matter.
4. d. All of the above.
5. c. Both Up Quarks and Down Quarks.
6. a. Quantum Mechanical Model.
7. d. Glucon.
8. a. W Bason.
9. b. Z Bason.
10. a. Protons.
11. c. Protons and Neutrons.
12. d. Neutrons.
13. a. Orbitals.
14. a. s
15. d. Spherical.
16. b. Bi-lobed.
17. b. Bi-lobed with a ring.
18. c. The Number of electrons is equal to the number of Protons.
19. b. Seven orbitals.
20. a. Linear Energy Transfer.
21. b. +2
22. a. -1
23. a. Quantum theory.
24. a. Electron Volt (eV)
25. a. Wave theory.
26. c. Tungsten.
27. a. 2mm;1 cm.
28. b. Focusing Cup.
29. a. Parabolic concave.
30. a. Oxidation.
31. d. 74
32. d. 3422-degree celcius.
33. c. 178 W m-1 k-1
34. c. Focal spot.
35. b. Effective Focal spot.
36. b. 20 degrees.
37. a. 1 x 3 mm.
38. a. 1 X 1 mm.
39. b. Focal track.
40. a. 100-500 milliamperes.
41. c. Cone Beam Units.
42. b. 3000 revolutions per minute.
43. a. 60 and 90 KVp.

44. c. 90-120 KVp.
45. a. Self rectified.
46. b. 60; 1/120 Second.
47. a. long contrast scale; Low dose to the Patient.
48. a. Number of Pulses/ Frequency of Power source.
49. c. 0.5 Second exposure.
50. b. Heat Units.
51. b. 20 KHU.
52. a. Tube rating.
53. b. Duty cycle.
54. c. 1: 60.
55. a. HU= Kvp x mA x seconds.
56. b. Hydrogen.
57. a. Radiation.
58. b. Radioactivity.
59. b. Hertzian waves.
60. d. Aluminum.
61. d. Copper.
62. d. Aluminum.
63. a. Collimator.
64. c. 7 cm.
65. a. Absorption interactions.
66. a. scattering interactions.
67. a. 90 % Absorbed; 10% Pass-through.
68. c. Compton scattering.
69. a. Coherent scattering.
70. a. Photoelectric absorption.
71. c. Third Power.
72. b. 6.5 Times.
73. a. Half value Layer.

Chapter 42

Radiation Units (Dosimetry)

Questions

1. The term Kerma is an acronym for the following?
    a. Kinetic energy radiated in mass.
    b. Kinetic energy is released in the matter.
    c. Kinetic energy radiated in the matter.
    d. Kinetic potential released in the matter.

2. These measures the capacity of x-rays to ionize air?
    a. Exposure.
    b. Kerma.
    c. Absorbed dose.
    d. Effective dose.

3. The dose is used to compare the biological effects of different types of radiation on a Tissue or organ.
    a. Absorbed dose.
    b. Equivalent dose.
    c. Effective dose.
    d. Kerma.

4. The following unit measures the intensity of radiation?
    a. Roentgen.
    b. Absorbed dose.
    c. Kerma.
    d. Equivalent dose.

5. The following unit is used to estimate the risk in Humans?
    a. Absorbed dose.
    b. Equivalent dose.
    c. Effective dose (E).
    d. Operator Accumulated dose.

6. The higher limits permitted for occupationally exposed persons?
   a. Operator Accumulated dose.
   b. Equivalent dose.
   c. Effective dose.
   d. Absorbed dose.

7. The International System of Units (SI) for Absorbed dose?
   a. Gray.
   b. Sievert.
   c. Air kerma.
   d. Becquerel.

8. The International System of Units (SI) for Radioactivity?
   a. Gray.
   b. Sievert.
   c. Becquerel.
   d. Air Kerma.

9. The International System of Units (SI) for Equivalent dose?
   a. Gray.
   b. Sievert.
   c. Air kerma.
   d. Becquerel.

10. The quantity of X-ray radiation through 0.00123 gram of air at 0 °C that produces ions in the air carrying one electrostatic unit of electric charge?
    a. Roentgen.
    b. Gray.
    c. Sievert.
    d. Air kerma.

11. The unit for measuring the radioactivity of a substance?
    a. Relative Biological Effectiveness (RBE).
    b. Operator Accumulated Dose (OAD).
    c. Effective dose.
    d. Equivalent dose.

12. The following is used to monitor the radiation exposure by a radiologist or radiographic Personnel operating in a radiation center?
    a. Thermoluminescent Dosimeter.
    b. Barometer.
    c. Thermography.
    d. Optical coherence Tomography.

13. The sum of the initial kinetic energies of all the charged particles liberated by uncharged ionizing radiation (neutrons and photons) in a sample of matter, divided by the mass of the sample material?
    a. Sievert.
    b. Kerma.
    c. Effective dose.
    d. Equivalent dose.

14. According to International Commission on Radiation Protection (ICRP), the annual occupational dose limit is?
    a. 50 mSv.
    b. 100 mSv.
    c. 150 mSv.
    d. 200 mSv.

15. The Maximum allowed dose to embryo or fetus during Pregnancy for radiation is?
    a. 0.5-1 mSv.
    b. 0.5-2 mSv.
    c. 2-3 mSv.
    d. 3-4 mSv.

16. The Maximum annual exposure limit for the Public for infrequent and continuous exposure to radiation according to the international commission on Radiation Protection (ICRP) and National Council on Radiation Protection and Measurements (NCRPM), respectively Is?
    a. five mSv and one mSv.
    b. two mSv and one mSv.
    c. three mSv and four mSv.
    d. four mSv and five mSv.

17. The mean skin exposure for one Periapical dental film is?
    a. 350 mR.
    b. 360 mR.
    c. 370 mR.
    d. 380 mR.

18. The effective dose for one radiation exposure by Panoramic Radiography is?
    a. 24 μSv.
    b. 25 μSv.
    c. 26 μSv.
    d. 27 μSv.

19. The effective dose for one radiation exposure by Computed Tomography of Maxilla?
    a. 104 to 1202 μSv.
    b. 204 to 1102 μSv.
    c. 304 to 1302 μSv.
    d. 404 to 1402 μSv.

20. The effective dose for one radiation exposure by Computed Tomography of Mandible?
    a. 561 to 2334 μSv.
    b. 661 to 3334 μSv.
    c. 761 to 3324 μSv.
    d. 861 to 3424 μSv.

21. The Thermoluminescent dosimeter used in radiology comprises the following ?
    a. Lithium Fluoride.
    b. Aluminium chloride.
    c. Barium Platinocyanide.
    d. Cellulose acetate.

22. Which of the following is not correct for Thermoluminescent Dosimeter?
    a. Must be worn below Lead apron by radiographic Personnel.
    b. Direct reading of radiation is impossible.
    c. The Thermoluminescent card reader is not essential.
    d. The readings are interpreted by Glow curve in a Thermoluminescent Card reader.

23. The production of 100 ergs of energy in one gram of tissue by any ionizing radiation?
    a. Radiation Absorbed Dose.
    b. Effective dose.
    c. Equivalent dose.
    d. Occupational accumulated dose.

Answers

1. b. Kinetic energy released in Matter.
2. b. Kerma.
3. b. Equivalent Dose.
4. a. Roentgen.
5. c. Effective dose.
6. a. Operator accumulated Dose.
7. a. Gray.
8. c. Becquerel.
9. b. Sievert.
10. a. Roentgen.
11. a. Relative Biological Effectiveness.
12. a. Thermoluminescent Dosimeter.
13. b. Kerma.
14. a. 50 mSv.
15. b. 0.5-2 mSv.
16. a. 5 mSv and 1 mSv.
17. b. 360 mSv.
18. c. 26μ Sv.
19. a. 104 –1202 μ Sv.
20. c. 761 – 3324 μ Sv.
21. a. Lithium Fluoride.
22. c. The Thermoluminescent card reader is not essential.
23. a. Radiation absorbed Dose.

Chapter 43

Radiation Biology

Questions

1. The study of the effects of ionizing radiation on living tissues?
   a. Radiation physics.
   b. Radiation Protection.
   c. Radiation Biology.
   d. Adsorption.

2. 2. The radiation effect in which a change is probable and does not have a threshold value is called?
   a. Stochastic effect.
   b. Deterministic effect.
   c. Compton effect.
   b. Photoelectric effect.

3. The radiation effect, which has a threshold dose and the severity of the response is proportional to the amount, is called?
   a. Stochastic effect.
   b. Deterministic effect.
   c. Photoelectric effect.
   d. Compton effect.

4. The following changes can occur inside the cell's nucleus by radiation except?
   a. Change of Nitrogenous base.
   b. Disruption of hydrogen bonds.
   c. Breakage of Hydrogen bonds.
   d. Addition of Nitrogenous bases.

5. The following changes can occur in the cell's cytoplasm after radiation exposure, except?
   a. Swelling of Mitochondria.
   b. Disorganization of Mitochondria.
   c. Focal necrosis.
   d. Decreased permeability to sodium and potassium ions.

6. The ability of the radiation to reduce the number of malignant cells below a critical level so that no further clinical manifestation of their presence will occur during the remaining time of the host is called?
   a. Radiocurability.
   b. Radioresponsiveness.
   c. Radiosensitivity.
   d. Stochastic effect.

7. The following are radioresistant except?
   a. Liposarcoma.
   b. osteosarcoma.
   c. Kaposi sarcoma.
   d. Myosarcoma.

8. The primary purpose of fractionation includes all the following except?
   a. Repair.
   b. Reoxygenation.
   c. Repopulation.
   d. Removal.

9. The ability of radiations to reduce the number of malignant cells below a critical level such that no further clinical manifestations of their presence will occur during the remaining lifetime of the host?
   a. Radioresponsiveness.
   b. Radiocurability.
   c. Radiosensitivity.
   d. Radioactivity.

10. The ability of radiations to biologically change the cells by killing or destroying their reproduction integrity?
    a. Radiosensitivity.
    b. Radiocurability.
    c. Radioresponsiveness.
    d. Radioactivity.

11. The time required for any changes to occur can be measured in the rate at which the clinical manifestations of radiation-induced biological evolution?
    a. Radiosensitivity.
    b. Radioresponsiveness.
    c. Radiocurability.
    d. Radioreactivity.

12. The following cells do not divide even in functional demand?
    a. Squamous epithelial cells.
    b. Basal cells of the oral mucous membrane.
    c. Parenchymal cells of salivary glands.
    d. Inner enamel epithelium of developing teeth.

13. The following cells divide regularly and are more radiosensitive?
    a. Basal cells of the oral mucous membrane.
    b. Inner enamel epithelium of developing teeth.
    c. Parenchymal cells of salivary glands.
    d. squamous epithelial cells.

14. The most sensitive period for inducing developmental abnormalities is during the following days of gestation?
    a. 18 to 45 days.
    b. 15 to 30 days.
    c. 20 to 40 days.
    d. 30 to 50 days.

15. Which of the following changes occur in saliva following radiation exposure of salivary glands?
    a. Decrease in Sodium, chloride, calcium, and Magnesium ions and Increased pH.
    b. Increase in sodium, chloride, calcium, and Magnesium ions and Decreased pH.
    c. Increase in Lubricating Properties.
    d. Atrophy of salivary glands.

Answers

1. c. Radiation Biology.
2. a. Stochastic effect.
3. b. Deterministic effect.
4. d. Addition of Nitrogenous Bases.
5. d. Decreased Permeability to Sodium and Potassium ions.
6. a. Radiocurability.
7. c. Kaposi sarcoma.
8. d. Removal.
9. b. Radiocurability.
10. a. Radiosensitivity.
11. b. Radioresponsiveness.
12. a. Squamous Epithelial cells.
13. a. Basal cells of the oral mucous membrane.
14. a. 18- 45 days.
15. b. Increase in sodium, chloride, calcium, magnesium ions, and decreased pH.

Chapter 44

Radiation Protection

Questions

1. According to the Position-Distance Rule, the operator must stand at these feet distance away from the source of radiation and at an angle to the direction of the central ray?
   a. 6 feet and 90° to 135°
   b. 7 feet and 90° to 150°
   c. 8 feet and 90° to 160°
   d. 9 feet and 90° to 170°

2. The reduction in Exposed Tissue Volume caused by Longer Focal Spot Film Distance?
   a. 12%
   b. 22%
   c. 32%
   d. 42%

3. The equipment operating at above 50 Kvp have a minimum distance from the end of the Position Indicating Device (PID) to the focal spot?
   a. 7 inches or 18 cm.
   b. 8 inches or 19 cm.
   c. 9 inches or 20 cm.
   d. 10 inches or 21 cm.

4. The diameter of the collimated X-ray Beam must be restricted to the following diameter at the Patient's Face?
   a. 2 ¾ inches.
   b. 3 ¾ inches.
   c. 4 ¾ inches.
   d. 5 ¾ inches.

5. Using an electronic timer permits exposure as low?
   a. 1/20 to 1/30 seconds.
   b. 1/ 30 to 1/40 seconds.
   c. 1/40 to 1/ 50 seconds.
   d. 1/50 to 1/60 seconds.

6. The thickness of the leaded Thyroid shield is?
   a. 0.1 mm.
   b. 0.2 mm.
   c. 0.3 mm.
   d. 0.4 mm.

7. What is the preferred concrete material used for shielding the x-ray room from radiation?
   a. Barium Plaster
   b. Gypsum.
   c. Dental stone.
   d. Bricks.

8. For proper shielding of the room from x-ray radiation, the concrete wall must be?
   a. 2"concrete, 1 mm Lead.
   b. 3"concrete, 1 mm Lead.
   c. 4"concrete, 2mm Lead.
   d. 5"concrete, 2 mm Lead.

9. To see the patient while being irradiated, the window must be such that it is not directed from the direction of the Primary Beam and must be made of the following material?
   a. Lead Glass.
   b. Silicate.
   c. Polythene.
   d. Bakelite.

10. The device used to measure the radiation exposure?
    a. Densitometer.
    b. Potentiometer.
    c. Ammeter.
    d. Voltmeter.

11. The indirect reading Dosimeter that needs frequent charging?
    a. Minometer.
    b. Densitometer.
    c. Potentiometer.
    d. Voltmeter.

12. The Dosimeter is sensitive only to high energy neutrons and hence used with other dosimeters?
    a. Pocket Dosimeter.
    b. Thermoluminescent Dosimeter.
    c. Track etch Dosimeter.
    d. Electronic Dosimeter.

13. The recommended wall thickness where the Primary and scattered x-rays fall must be, respectively?
    a. 35 cm and 23 cm.
    b. 45 cm and 33 cm.
    c. 55 cm and 43 cm.
    d. 65 cm and 53 cm.

14. The shielding in front of the doors and windows of the x-ray room is?
    a. 23 cm Brick Thickness or 1.7 mm Lead.
    b. 33 cm Brick Thickness or 1 mm Lead.
    c. 43 cm Brick Thickness or 2.7 mm Lead.
    d. 53 cm Brick Thickness or 3.7 mm Lead.

15. The minimum room size recommended for Dental radiography?
    a. 150 sq Feet.
    b. 200 Sq Feet.
    c. 250 sq Feet.
    d. 300 sq Feet.

16. The minimum space for Gantry of CT unit must not be less?
    a. 15 m^2
    b. 25 m^2
    c. 35 m^2
    d. 45 m^2

17. The safelight must be at the following distance from the processing tank surface?
    a. 1.2 m.
    b. 2.2 m.
    c. 3.2 m.
    d. 4.2 m.

Answers

1. a. 6 feet and 90-135°.
2. c. 32%.
3. a. 7 inches or 18 cm.
4. a. 2 ¾ inches.
5. a. 1/20 to 1/30 seconds.
6. b. 0.2 mm
7. a. Barium Plaster.
8. b. 3"concrete, 1 mm Lead.
9. a. Lead Glass.
10. b. Potentiometer.
11. a. Minometer.
12. c. Track etch Dosimeter.
13. a. 35 cm and 23 cm.
14. a. 23 cm Brick Thickness or 1. 7 mm Lead.
15. a. 150 sq Feet.
16. b. 25 m^2
17. a. 1.2 m.

Chapter 45

Radiographic Films

Questions

1. The size of the standard NO.2 adult size intraoral periapical radiographic film is?
   a. 21 X 25mm
   b. 31 x 41 mm
   c. 24 x 40mm
   d. 27 x 54 mm.

2. The size of the occlusal film used in dental radiography is?
   a. 55 x 65 mm.
   b. 57 x 76 mm.
   c. 58 x 77 mm.
   d. 59 x 78 mm.

3. The size of the film used for small children?
   a. 22 x 35 mm.
   b. 23 x 36mm.
   c. 24 x 37 mm.
   d. 25 x 38 mm.

4. The size of the OPG film is?
   a. 15 x 30 mm.
   b. 22 x 35 mm.
   c. 57 x 76 mm.

5. The following is a non-screen film?
   a. Intraoral Periapical radiograph.
   b. Orthopantomograph.
   c. Antero-posterior Skull view.
   d. Water's view.

6. Which of the following films has the highest speed?
   a. A speed.
   b. B speed.
   c. C speed.
   d. E speed.

7. The primary purpose of the lead foil in an intraoral periapical radiograph is?
   a. To prevent Backscattered radiation.
   b. To prevent contamination of saliva.
   c. To prevent contamination of processing solutions.
   d. To prevent light leaks.

8. The following film is single-coated?
   a. Intraoral periapical radiograph.
   b. Orthopantamograph.
   c. Occlusal radiograph.
   d. Mammography film.

9. The heart of the x-ray film is?
   a. Silver halide crystals in the emulsion layer.
   b. Protective outer base.
   c. Coating agents.
   d. Subcoat.

10. What is the primary purpose of the outermost plastic sheath in the intraoral periapical radiograph?
    a. To prevent ingress of saliva.
    b. To prevent light leaks.
    c. To prevent backscattered radiation.
    d. To provide rigidity to the film.

Answers

1. b. 31 X 41 mm.
2. b. 57 X 76 mm.
3. a. 22 X 35 mm.
4. a. 15 X 30 mm.
5. a. Intraoral Periapical radiograph.
6. d. E-Speed.
7. a. To prevent Backscattered radiation.
8. d. Mammography film.
9. a. Silver halide crystals in the emulsion layer.
10. a. To prevent ingress of saliva.

Chapter 46

Processing Solutions

Questions

1. The chemical constituent present in developer solution that serves as the first electron donor that converts silver ions to metallic silver at the latent image site is?
   a. Phenidone.
   b. Hydroquinone.
   c. sodium bicarbonate.
   d. Potassium bromide.

2. The developer solution for processing remains active only at a pH of about?
   a. 2
   b. 4
   c. 7
   d. 10

3. The activator present in the developer solution is?
   a. Sodium hydroxide.
   b. Potassium chloride.
   c. Calcium fluoride.
   d. Stannous fluoride.

4. The Preservative in the developer solution helps extend the shelf life?
   a. Sodium sulfite.
   b. Potassium bisulfite.
   c. Calcium carbonate.
   d. Sodium carbonate.

5. The following chemical ingredient in Developer acts as a restrainer and restrains the development of unexposed silver- halide grains?
   a. Calcium chloride.
   b. Stannous fluoride.
   c. Potassium bromide.
   d. Calcium fluoride.

6. The purpose of rinsing the radiographic film during processing is all EXCEPT?
   a. To dilute the Developer.
   b. slow the developing process.
   c. add the activator.
   d. Prevent neutralization of acid fixer.

7. The Purpose of Fixer in the radiographic film processing is all, EXCEPT?
   a. Removes developed silver halide crystals from the emulsion.
   b. hardens the emulsion.
   c. shrinks the emulsion.
   d. Removes undeveloped silver halide crystals from the emulsion.

8. The clearing agent present in the developer solution is?
   a. Hypo.
   b. Sodium fluoride.
   c. Sodium bicarbonate.
   d. Potassium fluoride.

9. The following chemical ingredient, acts as a preservative in Fixer, helps to prevent the oxidation of ammonium thiosulphate?
   a. Sodium hydroxide.
   b. Sodium carbonate.
   c. Ammonium sulfite.
   d. Potassium bromide.

10. The Hardener present in Fixer helps prevent damage to gelatin during subsequent handling and reduce swelling of the emulsion during the final wash?
    a. Aluminium sulfate.
    b. Potassium bromide.
    c. Calcium chloride.
    d. Sodium sulfite.

11. The recommended safelight filter used in the darkroom or safe room for processing radiographic films is called?
    a. Green GBX-2
    b. Red GBX-2
    c. Blue-GBX-2.
    d. yellow GBX-2.

12. The processing tank must be made of the following to prevent the corrosive action of chemicals?
    a. Stainless steel.
    b. Borosilicate.
    c. Bakelite.
    d. Polyethylene.

Answers

1. a. Phenidone.
2. d. 10
3. a. Sodium Hydroxide.
4. a. Sodium sulfite.
5. c. Potassium Bromide.
6. c. Add the activator.
7. d. Removes undeveloped silver halide crystals from the emulsion.
8. a. Hypo.
9. c. Ammonium Sulphite.
10. a. Aluminium sulfate.
11. b. Red GBX-2.
12. a. Stainless steel.

Chapter 47

Processing Errors

Questions

1. The appearance of terminal phalanges of either the patient's or dentist's finger in an intraoral periapical radiograph is called?
   a. Melanoma.
   b. Phalangioma.
   c. Xanthoma.
   d. Xanthelasma.

2. The fine black branched lines seen on the final processed radiographic image are due to the?
   a. A rapid removal of the film from the film packet.
   b. Slow removal of the film from film packet.
   c. Slow removal of the film from film packet.
   d. Medium speed removal of the film from film packet.

3. The Tyre track or Herringbone pattern is seen on the processed intraoral periapical radiograph is due to the?
   a. Correctly placed Intraoral periapical film before taking a radiograph.
   b. Reversely placed Intraoral periapical film before taking a radiograph.
   c. Improperly placed Intraoral periapical film before taking a radiograph.
   d. Upside down placement of Intraoral Periapical film before taking a radiograph.

4. When does the device's position indicating not adequately covering the intraoral film placed inside the oral cavity result in the following defect?
   a. Herringbone defect.
   b. Black branched lines.
   c. Cone cut image.
   d. White spots.

5. Can the following cause a yellow-brownish stain on the final processed intraoral periapical radiograph?
   a. Insufficient washing.
   b. Insufficient developing.
   c. Insufficient fixing.
   d. Movement of the patient.

6. The following contribute to film fog?
   a. Insufficient washing.
   b. Insufficient fixing.
   c. Insufficient developing.
   d. Improper safe lighting.

7. Why are the fine black branched lines in the processed radiographic film caused?
   a. Rapidity of removal of the radiographic film from Film packet.
   b. Slow removal of the radiographic film from film packet.
   c. Contamination of Developer.
   d. Contamination of Fixer.

8. The graininess in the film caused by extreme temperature changes in the developer and fixer solution is called?
   a. Static electricity.
   b. Reticulation.
   c. Dichroic fog.
   d. Anamnestic effect.

9. The double images on the processed radiograph are due?
   a. Double exposure.
   b. Reverse side placement of film.
   c. Contamination of fixer.
   d. Contamination of developer.

10. Blur on the processed radiograph is due?
    a. Patient movement during exposure.
    b. Restraining devices.
    c. A rapid removal of the film from the film packet.
    d. Contamination of developer and fixer.

Answers

1. b. Phalangioma.
2. a. Rapid removal of the film from film packet.
3. b. Reversely placed intraoral periapical film before taking a radiograph.
4. c. Cone cut image.
5. a. Insufficient Washing.
6. d. Improper safe lighting.
7. a. Rapidity of removal of the radiographic film from Film packet.
8. b. Reticulation.
9. a. Double exposure.
10. a. Patient movement during exposure.

Chapter 48

Radiographic Accessories

Questions

1. Do the Intensifying screens create an image receptor system that is more sensitive than film alone?
   a. 10 to 50 times.
   b. 5 to 50 times.
   c. 10 to 60 times.
   d. 10 to 70 times.

2. The intensifying screens are used in all the following Projections, EXCEPT?
   a. Panoramic projections.
   b. Cephalometric projections.
   c. Skull projections.
   d. Intraoral Periapical Projections.

3. The resolving power of intensifying screens is related to speed?
   a. Exponentially.
   b. Fractionally.
   c. Inversely proportional.
   d. Directly proportional.

4. The base in intensifying screen is?
   a. Polyester 0.25mm
   b. Polyethylene 0.25 mm
   c. Bakelite 0.25 mm.
   d. Phenidone 0.25 mm.

5. The intensifying screens contain phosphor layer, fluoresce green when absorbing x-ray photons?
   a. Yttrium tantalite.
   b. Beryllium iodide.
   c. Gadolinium oxysulphide.
   d. Cesium iodide.

6. The intensifying screens that fluoresce Blue by absorption of x-ray photons?
   a. Yttrium tantalite.
   b. Beryllium iodide.
   c. Gadolinium oxysulphide.
   d. Cesium iodide.

7. The blue-emitting phosphors in the intensifying screens are activated?
   a. Ruthenium.
   b. Barium.
   c. Niobium.
   d. Cesium.

8. The Green emitting phosphors in the intensifying screens are activated?
   a. Ruthenium.
   b. Terbium.
   c. Niobium.
   d. Caesium.

9. The following screen-film combinations are recommended for Dental extraoral diagnostics?
   a. 300 or faster.
   b. 400 or faster.
   c. 500 or faster.
   d. 600 or faster.

10. The emission spectrum from Lanex rare-earth intensifying screens peaks sharply at wavelength?
    a. 535nm.
    b. 545nm.
    c. 555nm.
    d. 565nm.

11. What are the Grids made?
    a. Alternate strips of Lead and Plastic.
    b. Alternate strips of Barium and Plastic.
    c. Alternate strips of Copper and Plastic.
    d. Alternate strips of Lead and Copper.

Answers

1. c. 10 to 60 times.
2. d. Intraoral Periapical Projections.
3. c. Inversely Proportional.
4. a. Polyester 0.25 mm.
5. c. Gadolinium oxysulphide.
6. a. Yttrium tantalate.
7. c. Niobium.
8. b. Terbium.
9. b. 400 or faster.
10. b. 545 nm.
11. a. Alternate strips of Lead and Plastic.

Chapter 49

Extraoral Imaging Techniques

Questions

1. The most common Extraoral radiographic techniques for assessing Facial asymmetry and assessment of orthognathic surgery outcomes involving maxillary, mandibular midline relationships?
   a. PA Cephalometric projection.
   b. Panoramic projections.
   c. Bitewing projections.
   d. Bisecting angle technique.

2. The Lefort fracture is often diagnosed by disturbances in the integrity of the following in a Panoramic image?
   a. Pterygomaxillary fissure.
   b. Superior orbital fissure.
   c. Inferior orbital fissure.
   d. Medial orbital fissure.

3. Ghost images are seen?
   a. Intraoral Periapical Film.
   b. Orthopantomographic Film.
   c. Occlusal Film.
   d. Laser Film.

4. The Extraoral radiographic techniques are indicated in the following conditions, EXCEPT?
   a. Severe Trismus.
   b. Evaluate skeletal Growth and Development.
   c. To examine the more considerable extent of odontogenic cysts and tumors.
   d. To evaluate periapical pathologies about maxillary and mandibular anterior teeth.

5. The following projection is called the occipitofrontal projection of the Nasal sinuses, excellent for evaluating the inner and middle ear region, especially frontal sinuses, anterior ethmoidal sinuses, and sphenoidal sinuses?
   a. Granger Projection.
   b. Submentovertex Projection.
   c. Towne's Projection.
   d. Reverse Towne's Projection.

6. The following extraoral projection is helpful for the evaluation of ethmoidal air cells and frontal sinus?
   a. Caldwell's Projection.
   b. Towne's Projection.
   c. Submentovertex Projection.
   d. Reverse Towne's Projection.

7. The following extraoral projection used to visualize fracture of coronoid process of mandible is?
   a. 30° Occipitomenton Projection (Modified Method).
   b. Towne's Projection.
   c. Submentovertex Projection.
   d. Granger Projection.

8. Is the following extraoral radiographic technique useful for visualizing fractures of the condylar neck region?
   a. Granger Projection.
   b. Water's Projection.
   c. Reverse Towne's Projection.
   d. Caldwell's Projection.

9. The following postauricular approach for directing the central ray used to evaluate the Lateral aspect of Temporomandibular joint space is called?
   a. Lindblom's technique.
   b. Grewcock approach.
   c. McQueen or Dell approach.
   d. Zimmer projection.

10. The extraoral radiographic technique used to visualize the anterior aspect of the Temporomandibular Joint space is?
    a. Granger Projection.
    b. Water's Projection.
    c. Zimmer Projection.
    d. McQueen or Dell approach.

11. The extraoral radiographic technique helps visualize sialolith within the Parotid gland?
    a. Topographic Mandibular occlusal radiographic projection.
    b. Granger Projection.
    c. Water Projection.
    d. Puffed cheek AP view.

Answers

1. a. P A Cephalometric Projection.
2. a. Pterygomaxillary fissure.
3. b. orthopantomographic Film.
4. d. To evaluate periapical pathologies about maxillary and mandibular anterior teeth.
5. a. Granger Projection.
6. a. Caldwell's Projection.
7. a. 30° Occipitomenton Projection (Modified Method).
8. c. Reverse Towne's Projection.
9. a. Lindblom's technique.
10. c. Zimmer's Projection.
11. d. Puffed cheek AP view.

Chapter 50

Intraoral Imaging Techniques

Questions

1. The best intraoral periapical imaging technique is?
   a. Bisecting angle technique.
   b. Short cone technique.
   c. Paralleling angle technique.
   d. Occlusal radiographic technique.

2. The technique of viewing the crowns of the maxillary and mandibular teeth and the alveolar crest on the same film?
   a. Bisecting angle technique.
   b. Short cone technique.
   c. Bitewing.
   d. Paralleling angle technique.

3. The technique that distorts the dentition is?
   a. Paralleling angle technique.
   b. Bisecting angle technique.
   c. Bitewing.
   d. Occlusal radiographic technique.

4. The technique used for detecting calculus deposits in interproximal areas is?
   a. Bisecting angle technique.
   b. Bitewing.
   c. Paralleling angle technique.
   d. Occlusal radiography.

5. The angulation of Position indicating device for Bitewing radiographic techniques?
    a. +5 degrees
    b. +10 degrees
    c. +15 degrees.
    d. +20 degrees.

6. The technique of placing a cotton roll on the palatal aspect of Maxillary molars before subjecting it to radiograph to prevent superimposition of the image of the zygomatic process of Maxilla over Maxillary posterior root is called?
    a. Le master's technique.
    b. Short cone technique.
    c. Long cone technique.
    d. Paralleling angle technique.

7. What is the intraoral radiographic technique used to detect whether an impacted tooth is buccally or lingually placed?
    a. Bisecting angle technique.
    b. Paralleling angle technique.
    c. Orthopantomography.
    d. Occlusal radiographic Projections.

8. The following image receptor is more suitable and comfortable for imaging dentition among the pediatric population?
    a. Digital sensors.
    b. Paralleling angle technique.
    c. Occlusal radiographic Projections.
    d. Lateral cephalometric Projections.

9. The following radiographic technique helps locate sialolith?
    a. Bisecting angle technique.
    b. Paralleling angle technique.
    c. Lateral Cephalometric Projection.
    d. Mandibular occlusal radiograph.

10. Is the intraoral radiographic technique best for assessing the periapical status of teeth?
    a. Occlusal radiography.
    b. Bitewing radiograph.
    c. Paralleling angle technique.
    d. Bisecting angle technique.

11. The Bisecting angle technique is based on the following rule?
    a. Ciesenzky's rule of isometry.
    b. Buccal-object rule.
    c. Gill's approach.
    d. Grewcut approach.

12. What is the intraoral radiographic technique that helps localize whether the impacted tooth is buccally or palatally placed?
    a. Ciesenzky's rule of isometry.
    b. Clark's technique.
    c. Grewcut approach.
    d. Lindblom's technique.

13. The technique in which one intraoral periapical and an occlusal radiograph is taken in the same anatomical region for the location of the impacted tooth?
    a. Miller's right-angle technique.
    b. Clark's technique.
    c. Lindblom's technique.
    d. Gill's approach.

14. The technique based on beam direction rather than tube direction is?
    a. Richard's technique.
    b. Clark's technique.
    c. Lindblom's technique.
    d. Miller's right angle technique.

Answers

1. c. Paralleling angle Technique.
2. c. Bitewing.
3. a. Paralleling angle technique.
4. b. Bitewing.
5. b. +10 Degrees.
6. a. Le master's technique.
7. d. Occlusal radiographic technique.
8. a. Digital sensors.
9. d. Mandibular occlusal radiograph.
10. c. Paralleling angle Technique.
11. a. Ciesenzky's rule of isometry.
12. b. Clark's technique.
13. a. Miller's right angle technique.
14. a. Richard's technique.

Chapter 51

Orthopantamography

Questions

1. The following are the characteristics of Ghost Image in an orthopantomography, EXCEPT?
   a. Always appear on the same side of the actual anatomical location.
   b. Appears Higher level.
   c. Appears blurred mesiodistally.
   d. Appears enlarged superior-inferiorly than mesiodistally.

2. The anteroposterior positioning of the patient is achieved by placing the patient's Maxillary and mandibular incisors on a notched positioning device called?
   a. True block.
   b. Twin block.
   c. Bite block.
   d. Anatomical block.

3. The following are the advantages of orthopantomography, EXCEPT?
   a. Less coverage of Facial bones and teeth.
   b. It can be used in patients with trismus.
   c. It can be used in patients who are not able to tolerate IOPA.
   d. Aid in Patient education.

4. The following are the indications of Panoramic radiography, EXCEPT?
   a. Overall Evaluation of dentition.
   b. Gross Evaluation of TMJ.
   c. Evaluate the position of affected teeth.
   d. Evaluate periapical lesion in the maxillary and mandibular anterior region.

5. The main disadvantages of Orthopantomography include the following, EXCEPT?
   a. Do not provide fine details compared to Intraoral Periapical radiographs.
   b. Requires accurate positioning to avoid positioning errors and artifacts.
   c. Difficult to image in patients with severe maxillomandibular discrepancy.
   d. Difficult and inconvenient radiographic Technique.

6. The following are true about ghost images except?
   a. Always seen on the opposite side.
   b. Placed at a higher position than the opposite original counterpart.
   c. Appear blur mesiodistally and clearer supero-inferiorly.
   d. Always seen on the same side.

7. The three-dimensional curvilinear zone in which the object placed appears in the final radiograph?
   a. Focal spot.
   b. Focal zone.
   c. Focal trough.
   d. Focal area.

8. The radiographic technique of choice when one cannot open the mouth due to severe trismus?
   a. Orthopantomograph.
   b. Occlusal radiograph.
   c. Bitewing radiograph.
   d. Intraoral periapical radiograph.

9. The following radiograph provides a gross overall detail of the dentition status, such as whether a tooth is under eruption or impacted?
   a. Occlusal radiography.
   b. Orthopantomography.
   c. Bitewing radiograph.
   d. Ultrasonography.

10. The following areas usually appear blurred in orthopantomography due to superimposition of the cervical spine?
    a. Maxillary and mandibular incisor and Lateral incisor region.
    b. Maxillary and mandibular premolar and molar region.
    c. Mandibular premolar and molar region.
    d. Maxillary and mandibular canine region.

Answers

1. a. Always appear on the same side of its actual anatomic location.
2. c. Bite Block.
3. a. Less coverage of Facial Bones and teeth.
4. d. Evaluate Periapical lesion in Maxillary and Mandibular anterior region.
5. d. Difficult and inconvenient radiographic Technique.
6. d. Always seen on the same side.
7. c. Focal trough.
8. a. Orthopantomograph.
9. b. Orthopantomography.
10. a. Maxillary and mandibular incisor and lateral incisor region.

Chapter 52

Digital Imaging

Questions

1. The Photostimulable Phosphor Plates comprise?
   a. Gadolinium doped with Barium fluorohalide.
   b. Chromium doped with Barium fluorohalide.
   c. Europium doped with Barium fluorohalide.
   d. Selenium doped with Barium fluorohalide.

2. The Photostimulable Phosphor Plates are more sensitive?
   a. Red light spectrum.
   b. Greenlight spectrum.
   c. Violet light spectrum.
   d. Yellow light spectrum.

3. A type of high-frequency noise characterized by isolated small regions surrounded by lighter or darker regions is called?
   a. Speckling.
   b. Despeckling.
   c. Auto filters.
   d. Semiauto filters.

4. The filters that remove high-frequency noise smoothen the image is called?
   a. Speckling.
   b. Despeckling filters.
   c. Auto filters.
   d. Semiauto filters.

5. The process by which Filters sharpen the image by either removing low-frequency noise or enhancing boundaries between images with different intensities is called?
   a. Edge enhancement.
   b. Speckling.
   c. Despeckling.
   d. Auto filters.

6. The purpose of reducing file size with critical image preservation is called?
   a. DeCompression.
   b. Compression.
   c. Speckling.
   d. Edge enhancement.

7. The acceptable compression rate for evaluating image quality objectively and detecting artificial lesions in Panoramic radiographs?
   a. 12:1
   b. 15:1
   c. 25:1
   d. 28:1

8. The term JPEG which provides a range of compression of photographs, stands for?
   a. Joint Peak Photographic Energy Group.
   b. Joint Photographic Experts Group.
   c. Joint Peak Energy Group.
   d. Joint Photographic Energy Group.

9. The agent of choice for disinfection of digital image receptors is?
   a. Wiping with Isopropyl alcohol.
   b. Immersing in Isopropyl alcohol.
   c. Immersing in Gluteraldehyde.
   d. Immersing in Sodium hypochlorite.

10. The following were the drawbacks of Photostimulable phosphor plates, EXCEPT?
    a. Inability to distinguish images from plates exposed backward.
    b. Inability to sterilize by heat.
    c. Longer scanning time.
    d. Rigid does not fracture.

11. Which of the following sensor has the property of erase-memory?
    a. CMOS.
    b. CCD.
    c. PSP.
    d. CID.

Answers

1. c. Europium doped with Barium fluorohalide.
2. a. Red Light Spectrum.
3. a. Speckling.
4. b. Despeckling filters.
5. a. Edge enhancement.
6. b. Compression.
7. d. 28:1.
8. b. Joint Photographic Experts Group.
9. a. Wiping with Isopropyl alcohol.
10. d. Rigid does not fracture.
11. c. PSP

Chapter 53

Temporomandibular Joint Imaging

Questions

1. The technique of viewing medial aspect of Temporomandibular Joint?
   a. Transcranial.
   b. Grewcock approach.
   c. Transpharyngeal view.
   d. Lindblom's Technique.

2. The technique of viewing the anterior aspect of the Temporomandibular Joint?
   a. Zimmer's view.
   b. Mcqueen's view.
   c. Infra-cranial Projection.
   d. Pharma Projection.

3. The technique of visualizing lateral aspect of Temporomandibular Joint?
   a. Zimmer's view.
   b. Pharma Projection.
   c. Grewcut approach.
   d. Infra-cranial Projection.

4. The following is used to compare the extent of condylar movement in open and closed mouth positions?
   a. Temporomandibular Joint Tomography.
   b. Mc Queen's Projection.
   c. Lindblom's Technique.
   d. Orthopantomography.

5. The characteristic obliteration of interarticular space is seen?
   a. Bony Ankylosis.
   b. Effusion of Temporomandibular joint.
   c. Osteosarcoma affecting condyle.
   d. Fibrinous adhesions of the articular disc.

6. The technique of visualizing the Temporomandibular joint by placing behind half an inch below the posterior auricular region is?
   a. Grewcut approach.
   b. Zimmer's projection.
   c. Mc Queen's projection.
   d. Dell projection.

7. The temporomandibular joint projection with a high cataract formation incidence?
   a. Zimmer's projection.
   b. Lindblom's technique.
   c. Gill's approach.
   d. Grewcut approach.

8. The technique of imaging the Temporomandibular joint in which the point of the central ray is directed half an inch behind and 2 inches above external acoustic meatus?
   a. Lindblom's technique.
   b. Gille's approach.
   c. Grewcock approach.
   d. Zimmer's projection.

9. The radiographic view used to visualize fracture of the condylar neck?
   a. Reverse Towne's view.
   b. Zimmer's view.
   c. Lindblom's technique.
   d. Gille's approach.

10. The technique used for visualizing the occipital areas of the skull?
    a. Towne's projection.
    b. Lindblom's technique.
    c. Gill's approach.
    d. Mc queen Dell projection.

Answers

1. c. Transpharyngeal view.
2. a. Zimmer's view.
3. c. Grewcut approach.
4. a. Temporomandibular Joint Tomography.
5. a. Bony Ankylosis.
6. a. Grewcut approach.
7. a. Zimmer's Projection.
8. a. Lindblom's technique.
9. a. Reverse Towne's view.
10. a. Towne's projection.

Chapter 54

Contrast Mediums in Imaging

Questions

1. The contrast medium used in Computed Tomography?
   a. Iodine.
   b. Gadolinium.
   c. Lipiodol.
   d. Iopamate.

2. The contrast medium used for imaging the adrenal medulla (Phaeochromocytoma) tumors?
   a. MIBG.
   b. Iodine.
   c. Lipiodol.
   d. Iopamate.

3. The contrast agent used for determining the progression and monitoring atherosclerotic plaques in coronary arteries?
   a. MIBG.
   b. Iodine.
   c. Europium doped with small superparamagnetic iron oxide particles (Eu-VSOP)
   d. Iohexol.

4. The time taken by a normal functioning kidney takes these hours for clearing contrast medium from the body?
   a. Approximately 10 hours.
   b. Approximately 20 Hours.
   c. Approximately 30 Hours.
   d. Approximately 40 Hours.

5. The contrast medium of choice in Nuclear Magnetic Spectroscopy?
   a. Hyperpolarized ^{13}C.
   b. Gadolinium.
   c. Iodine.
   d. Pantopaque.

6. The more stable Gadolinium contrast agent in MRI?
   a. Gadoteridol.
   b. Gadopentetate Dimeglumine.
   c. Gadoversetamide.
   d. Gadodiamide.

7. What is the most common adverse effect after intravenous infusion of Gadolinium-based contrast agents?
   a. Nephrogenic systemic Fibrosis.
   b. Dermatitis.
   c. Alopecia.
   d. Pruritis.

8. The contrast agent likely to accumulate in the dentate nucleus of the Brain?
   a. Pantopaque.
   b. Iodine.
   c. Gadolinium-based contrast agents.
   d. Hyperpolarized ^{13}C

9. The contrast agent with a linear Ligand?
   a. Diethylenetriaminepentaaceticacid (DTPA) in Gadopentetate dimeglumine.
   b. Gadoteridol.
   c. Gadodiamide.
   d. Gadoversetamide.

10. The contrast medium used in CT imaging?
    a. Iodine.
    b. Gadoteridol.
    c. Pantopaque.
    d. Diethylenetriaminepentaaceticacid (DTPA).

Answers

1. a. Iodine.
2. a. MIBG.
3. c. Europium doped with small superparamagnetic iron oxide particles (Eu-VSOP)
4. b. Approximately 20 hours.
5. a. Hyperpolarized ^{13}C.
6. a. Gadoteridol.
7. a. Nephrogenic Systemic Fibrosis.
8. c. Gadolinium-based contrast agents.
9. a. Diethylenetriaminepentaaceticacid (DTPA) in Gadopentetate dimeglumine.
10. a. Iodine.

Chapter 55

Ultrasonography

Questions

1. The wavelength of the ultrasound is?
   a. 1500 to 20,000Hz
   b. Above 20,000 Hz
   c. 10,000 to 20,000 Hz
   d. 1500 to 10,000 Hz

2. The transducer in ultrasonography comprises?
   a. Lead zirconate titanate.
   b. Barium fluorohalide.
   c. cesium iodide.
   d. Calcium fluoride.

3. Does the absence of the following bone on ultrasonographic imaging during the first trimester of Pregnancy (11th-14th weeks of gestation) help diagnose Down syndrome?
   a. Nasal Bone
   b. Maxilla
   c. Mandible
   d. Vertebrae.

4. The ultrasound signal transmitted into a patient gets attenuated by all the following, EXCEPT?
   a. Diffusion.
   b. Reflection.
   c. Absorption.
   d. Deflection.

5. The recent ultrasound techniques have transducers that allow echoes to be processed at a rapid rate to allow motion perception is called?
   a. Real-time imaging.
   b. Fusion imaging.
   c. Diffusion-weighted imaging.
   d. Auto imaging.

6. The tissues that do not produce signals are said to be Anechoic?
   a. Fluid-filled cysts.
   b. Needle.
   c. Ligaments.
   d. Skin.

7. The following imaging is used for the evaluation of blood flow?
   a. Colour doppler ultrasound.
   b. Ultrasound.
   c. Computed Tomography.
   d. Occlusal radiography.

8. The current ultrasonographic techniques allow echoes to be processed at a sufficiently rapid rate to enable the perception of motion referred?
   a. Real-time imaging.
   b. Confocal spectroscopy.
   c. Myelography.
   d. Filmless imaging.

9. The frequency of ultrasound probes used for imaging salivary glands?
   a. 2.5-4 MHz.
   b. 7.5-18 MHz.
   c. 1-3 MHz.
   d. 24-28 MHz.

10. Ultrasonography is helpful in the following EXCEPT?
    a. To differentiate solid and cystic lesions.
    b. To study salivary gland tumors.
    c. Do not cause damage to tissue by ionization.
    d. Poor resolution and hence more operator dependent.

Answers

1. a. 1,500-20,000 Hz.
2. a. Lead Zirconate Titanate.
3. a. Nasal Bone.
4. d. Deflection.
5. a. Real-Time imaging.
6. a. Fluid-filled cysts.
7. a. Colour Doppler Ultrasound.
8. a. fluid-filled cysts.
9. b. 7.5-18 MHz.
10. c. Do not cause damage to live tissue by ionization.

Chapter 56

Contrast Imaging Techniques

Questions

1. The technique of visualizing and studying the ductal architecture of the salivary gland by radiographic infusion of Contrast medium into the duct is called?
   a. Fluoroscopy.
   b. Sialography.
   c. Sialendoscopy.
   d. Spectroscopy.

2. The technique of visualizing the sialolith under the guidance of fiber optic cable with an intraoral camera attached at its tip is?
   a. Fluoroscopy.
   b. Sialendoscopy.
   c. Spectroscopy.
   d. Lymphangiography.

3. The technique of studying the lymphatic vessels and their architectural variations by infusion of radiographic contrast medium into the lymphatic vessels?
   a. Fluoroscopy.
   b. Sialendoscopy.
   c. Spectroscopy.
   d. Lymphangiography.

4. Percutaneous Baloon vascular decompression for relieving superior cerebellar artery vascular compression on Trigeminal ganglion is done under the guidance?
   a. Fluoroscopy.
   b. Spectroscopy.
   c. Lymphangiography.
   d. Sialography.

5. The technique of identifying brain tumors by analyzing the chemical constituents like choline is called?
   a. MR Spectroscopy.
   b. Sialography.
   c. Fluoroscopy.
   d. Lymphangiography.

6. The technique for visualizing the vascular indentations by looping the superior cerebellar artery in Trigeminal neuralgia?
   a. MR Angiography.
   b. Myelography.
   c. Lymphangiography.
   d. Ventilation Perfusion scan.

7. A Ventilation Perfusion scan is used to detect?
   a. Pulmonary nodule.
   b. Pulmonary embolism.
   c. Calcified Pulmonary lymph node.
   d. Pleural effusion.

8. The imaging technique used for images of CSF and hence valuable for the diagnosis of CSF rhinorrhea?
   a. Cisternography.
   b. Ureterography.
   c. Angiography.
   d. Lymphangiography.

9. The technique of introducing a contrast medium around the spinal canal to study the subarachnoid space is called?
   a. Myelography.
   b. Lymphangiography.
   c. Ureterography.
   d. Sialography.

10. What is the jet phenomenon seen in barium swallow because of the oesophageal web?
    a. Plummer-Vinson syndrome.
    b. Marfan syndrome.
    c. Down syndrome.
    d. Mc Cune Albright syndrome.

11. The real-time intraoperative detection of bone metastasis, bone growth, and tissue microcalcification?
    a. Near-infrared fluorescence imaging.
    b. Tuned aperture computed tomography.
    c. Subtraction radiography.
    d. Fluoroscopy.

Answers

1. b. Sialography.
2. b. Sialendoscopy.
3. d. Lymphangiography.
4. a. Fluoroscopy.
5. a. MR Spectroscopy.
6. a. MR angiography.
7. b. Pulmonary embolism.
8. a. Cisternography.
9. a. Myelography.
10. a. Plummer Vinson syndrome.
11. a. Near-infrared fluorescence imaging.

Chapter 57

Computed Tomography

Questions

1. The Computer Tomography was invented?
   a. Sir Godfrey Hounsfield
   b. Paul brucella
   c. Metchnikoff
   d. Albert Edison

2. The Computed Tomography imaging was first introduced in the year?
   a. 1970
   b. 1971
   c. 1972
   d. 1973

3. The shape of the x-ray beam produced by Computed Tomography is?
   a. Fan-shaped beam.
   b. Cone-shaped beam.
   c. Spherical-shaped beam.
   d. Rectangular-shaped beam.

4. The CT scanners in which patients lie on a stationary table while the x-ray source rotates one cycle around them, after which the table moves 1-5mm for the following scan is called?
   a. Incremental scanners.
   b. Prepositional scanners.
   c. Positional scanners.
   d. Orthogonal scanners.

5. The formula gives the Pitch in CT?
   a. Pitch = Table travel per x-ray tube rotation/ Image thickness.
   b. Pitch = Image thickness/ Table travel per x-ray tube rotation.
   c. Pitch = Image thickness/ Table thickness.
   d. Pitch = Table thickness/ Image Thickness.

6. The MDCT scanners were introduced during the year?
   a. 1996
   b. 1997
   c. 1998
   d. 1999

7. In MDCT, the following number of detector arrays are used with a helical CT scanner?
   a. 64 or 128.
   b. 54 or 118.
   c. 44 or 108.
   d. 34 or 108.

8. The time for MDCT to make a complete cycle around the patient?
   a. 0.15 second.
   b. 0.25 second.
   c. 0.35 second.
   d. 0.45 second.

9. The CT scanners operate at these parameters?
   a. 80-140kVp, 200-800mA, 0.5-2.0mm
   b. 60-120kVp, 100-700Ma, 0.1-2.0mm
   c. 50-120kVp, 100-700mA, 1.0-2.0 mm
   d. 40-110kVp, 100-600mA, 1.0-2.0mm

10. The slice thickness in MDCT is?
    a. 1-2 mm.
    b. 1-3 mm.
    c. 1-4mm.
    d. 1-5mm.

11. The detectors in MDCT comprise?
    a. Sio2.
    b. Gd2 S2o.
    c. Cs2 s20.
    d. Ps2S20.

12. The individual Pixels in MDCT are about the following dimension?
    a. 0.525 mm.
    b. 0.625 mm.
    c. 0.725 mm.
    d. 0.825 mm.

13. The length of the voxel in MDCT is?
    a. 1-5 mm.
    b. 1-10mm.
    c. 1-20mm.
    d. 1-30mm.

14. The reconstruction algorithm used to reconstruct images in MDCT is?
    a. Feldkamp algorithm.
    b. Fournier algorithm.
    c. Gasson algorithm.
    d. Projection algorithm.

15. The filters used to minimize the noise in low-contrast objects such as soft tissue is called?
    a. Smoothing Filters.
    b. Edge -sharpening filters.
    c. Despeckling filters.
    d. Back-projection filters.

16. The filters used to improve visualization of fine bony detail is called?
    a. Edge -sharpening filters.
    b. Smoothing filters.
    c. Back-projection filters.
    d. Despeckling filters.

17. The Hounsfield units for water is?
    a. 0
    b. +10
    c. +20
    d. +30

18. The image optimized for viewing bone may have a window width?
    a. 700 units.
    b. 600 units.
    c. 500 units.
    d. 400 units.

19. The image optimized to view soft tissues may have a window width?
    a. 400 units.
    b. 300 units.
    c. 200 units.
    d. 100 units.

20. The Main advantages of CT over conventional film radiography include EXCEPT?
    a. Eliminating structures inside the area of interest.
    b. Inherent high contrast resolution.
    c. Can distinguish differences between adjacent tissues that differ in physical density less than 1%.
    d. Multiplanar reformatted imaging is possible.

21. The process of three-dimensional reformatting requires that each original voxel, shaped as a rectangular solid, be dimensionally altered into multiple cuboidal voxels called?
    a. Interpolation.
    b. Transformation.
    c. Reformatting.
    d. Manipulation.

22. The artifact that results because of voxel having finite dimensions. When a voxel has both tissues (soft tissue and hard), the resulting CT number for that voxel is an intermediate value that does not represent either tissue. The resulting image may be blurring the junction of tissues or losing part of a thin cortical layer of bone?
    a. Partial volume artifact.
    b. Cone-beam effect.
    c. Beam hardening artifact.
    d. Metal streaking artifact.

23. The artifact that can occur in CT due to preferential absorption of lower energy photons in the heterogeneous x-ray beam is called?
    a. Partial volume artifact.
    b. Cone-beam effect.
    c. Beam hardening artifact.
    d. Metal streaking artifact.

24. The artifact that occurs due to near-complete absorption of x-ray photons by metallic restorations appears as radiopaque streaks in the occlusal plane?
    a. Partial volume artifact.
    b. Cone -beam effect.
    c. Beam hardening artifact.
    d. Metal streaking artifact.

25. The technology in which helical acquisition is made possible in computed tomography scanners?
    a. slip-ring technology.
    b. nonslip-ring technology.
    c. stationary-ring technology.
    d. moving-ring technology.

26. What is a dimensionless quantity used to express a linear transformation of the measured attenuation coefficient in a simple number in Computed Tomography Imaging?
    a. Hounsfield unit.
    b. standardised unit.
    c. International unit.
    d. Standard International unit.

27. The Hounsfield unit value of air in CT imaging?
    a. + 60
    b. - 100
    c. - 1000
    d. +2500

28. The first-generation CT scanner had the following number of detectors?
    a. 1-2
    b. 3-4
    c. 4-5
    d. 5-6

29. The fourth-generation CT scanners have more than the following number of detectors in the outer ring fixed?
    a. 500
    b. 1000
    c. 2000
    d. 3000

30. The first-generation CT scanner has the following x-ray beam?
    a. Pencil -like
    b. Arc-like
    c. Fan-like
    d. Circular-like

31. The scintillation detector in a CT scan comprises?
    a. Potassium iodide
    b. Magnesium iodide
    c. Caesium iodide
    d. Barium iodide

32. In a single slice CT, the table distance traveled in one 360° gantry rotation divided by beam collimation?
    a. Detector Pitch
    b. Gantry Pitch.
    c. Crouch Pitch
    d. Beam Pitch

33. The following Pitch values result in more excellent image quality but increased Patient dose?
    a. <1
    b. ≥ 1
    c. $=1$
    d. ≤ 1

34. In a Multislice CT scan, the table distance traveled in one 360° gantry rotation divided by the total thickness of all simultaneously acquired slices is called?
    a. Beam Pitch
    b. Detector Pitch
    c. Gantry Pitch
    d. Crouch Pitch

Answers

1. a. Sir Godfrey Hounsfield.
2. a. 1970
3. a. Fan-shaped x-ray beam.
4. a. Incremental scanners.
5. a. Pitch = Table travel per x-ray tube rotation/ Image thickness.
6. c. 1998.
7. a. 64 or 128.
8. b. 0.25 seconds.
9. a. 80-140kVp, 200-800mA, 0.5-2.0mm
10. b. 1-3 mm.
11. b. Gd2 s20
12. b. 0.625 mm.
13. c. 1-20 mm.
14. a. Feldkamp algorithm.
15. a. Smoothing filters.
16. a. Edge sharpening filters.
17. a. 0
18. a. 700 units.
19. a. 400 units.
20. a. The elimination of structures inside the area of interest.
21. a. Interpolation.
22. a. Partial volume artifact.
23. c. Beam hardening artifact.
24. d. Metal streaking artifact.
25. a. Slip ring technology.
26. a. Hounsfield units.
27. c. - 1000
28. a. 1-2
29. d. 3000
30. a. Pencil-like.
31. c. Cesium iodide.
32. a. Detector Pitch.
33. a. < 1.
34. a. Beam Pitch.

Chapter 58

Magnetic Resonance Imaging

Questions

1. The technique of imaging without ionizing radiation?
   a. Computed Tomography.
   b. Magnetic resonance imaging.
   c. Cone-beam computed Tomography.
   d. Orthopantomography

2. Which of the specialized imaging modality is very noisy?
   a. Computed Tomography.
   b. Magnetic resonance imaging.
   c. Orthopantomography.
   d. Cone-beam computed Tomography.

3. Nuclear Magnetic resonance was discovered?
   a. Felix Bloch and Edward Mills Purcell.
   b. Hounsfield
   c. Paul bunnet
   d. Miller

4. The coils used to produce deliberate variations in the main magnetic field in Magnetic Resonance Imaging are called?
   a. Gradient coil
   b. Phased array coil
   c. Surface coil
   d. Radiofrequency coil

5. The Gradient coils in Magnetic Resonance Imaging for magnetic field variations along the z-axis are called?
   a. Helmholtz Pairs
   b. Saddle coils
   c. Phased array coil
   d. Radiofrequency coil

6. The Gradient coils in Magnetic Resonance Imaging for providing variations in a magnetic field along the x and y-axis are called?
   a. saddle coils
   b. Helmholtz pairs
   c. Radiofrequency coil
   d. Phased array coil.

7. These coils receive only the radiofrequency signals in Magnetic Resonance Imaging?
   a. Phased array coil
   b. Radiofrequency coil
   c. Saddle coil
   d. Helmholtz Pairs

8. These coils are a loop of circular or rectangular wire and placed over the region of interest?
   a. surface coil.
   b. Paired saddle coil.
   c. Birdcage coil.
   d. Helmholtz Pair coil

9. The following coil is used for imaging small body parts such as the Temporomandibular Joint?
   a. Surface coil.
   b. Paired saddle coil.
   c. Helmholtz pair coil.
   d. Birdcage coil.

10. The following coil provides the best Radiofrequency Homogeneity of all the radiofrequency coils?
    a. Surface coil.
    b. Paired saddle coil.
    c. Helmholtz pair coil.
    d. Birdcage coil.

11. The radiofrequency transceiver coil used for imaging of the head?
    a. surface coil.
    b. Paired saddle coil.
    c. Helmholtz pair coil.
    b. Birdcage coil.

12. The portion of the gradient coils and the associated current perpendicular to the main magnetic field causes a force on the coils called?
    a. Lorentz force
    b. Dipole force
    c. Quantum force
    d. Swivel force

13. In Magnetic resonance Imaging, the spin magnetization vector precesses (rotates) around the magnetic field at a frequency called?
    a. Larmour frequency.
    b. Spatial frequency.
    c. Quantum frequency.
    d. Dipole frequency.

14. The metalloporphyrin commonly used as a contrast agent in Magnetic Resonance imaging is?
    a. Manganese (III) tetra- [4- sulfanatophenyl] porphyrin
    b. Calcium (III) tetra-[4-sulfanatophenyl] porphyrin
    c. Ruthenium(III) tetra-[4-sulfanatophenyl] porphyrin
    d. Rubidium(III) tetra-[4-sulfanatophenyl] porphyrin

15. If used in Nuclear Magnetic Resonance imaging, the nitroxide contrast agent can be immediately reversed by intravenous injection?
    a. Sodium ascorbate
    b. Ferrous ascorbate
    c. Calcium ascorbate
    d. Magnesium ascorbate

16. The superparamagnetic iron oxide consists of nanoparticles of iron oxide crystals coated in carbohydrates and used to treat iron-deficiency anemia in patients with chronic kidney disease?
    a. Ferrochrome
    b. Ferumoxytol
    c. Ferrozinc
    d. Ferroferrin

17. The nuclear magnetic resonance technique that allows tissues to be interrogated for the presence and concentration of various metabolites?
    a. Nuclear Magnetic Resonance.
    b. Magnetic Resonance Spectroscopy.
    c. Computed Tomography.
    d. Cone Beam computed Tomography.

18. The imaging technique that helps assess the grading of tumors of the brain?
    a. Nuclear Magnetic Resonance
    b. Magnetic Resonance Spectroscopy.
    c. Computed Tomography
    d. Cone Beam computed Tomography

19. The following metabolite changes occur in Nuclear Magnetic Resonance as the grading of tumors increases?
    a. Increase in Choline, Lipids, Lactate, and Decrease in creatine
    b. Decrease in choline, Lipids, Lactate, and Increase in creatine
    c. Decrease in choline, Lipids, Lactate, and Decrease in creatine.
    d. Increase in choline, Lipids, Lactate, and Increase in creatine.

20. The metabolite increased in Nuclear magnetic Resonance imaging is?
    a. Choline.
    b. Lactate.
    c. Lipid.
    d. Creatine.

Answers

1. b. Magnetic Resonance Imaging.
2. b. Magnetic Resonance Imaging.
3. a. Felix Bloch and Edward Mills Purcell.
4. a. Gradient coils.
5. a. Helmholtz Pairs.
6. a. Paired saddle coils.
7. b. Radiofrequency coils.
8. a. Surface coils.
9. a. Surface coil.
10. c. Helmholtz Pair coil.
11. d. Birdcage coil.
12. a. Lorentz force.
13. a. Larmour frequency.
14. a. Manganese (III) Tetra-[4-Sulphanatophenyl Porphyrin.
15. d. Magnesium ascorbate.
16. b. Ferumoxytol.
17. b. Magnetic Resonance spectroscopy.
18. b. Magnetic Resonance spectroscopy.
19. a. Increase in choline, lipids, Lactate, decrease in creatine
20. a. Choline.

Chapter 59

MRI Artifacts

Questions

1. A type of MRI artifact where one or more spurious bands of electronic noise extend perpendicular to the frequency encode direction and present in all series images?
   a. Zipper artifact
   b. Herringbone artifact
   c. Starry sky artifact
   d. Wrap around artifact

2. An MRI artifact related to one or few aberrant data point(s) in k-space caused by fluctuating power supply resulting in discrepancy in Radiofrequency Pulses?
   a. Corduroy artifact
   b. Wrap-around artifact
   c. Starry sky artifact.
   d. Zipper artifact

3. The appearance of alternate bright and dark bands in an MRI image is called?
   a. Zebra stripes
   b. Wrap around artifact
   c. starry sky artifact
   d. Zipper artifact

4. The interference pattern is most commonly seen when acquiring gradient-echo images using the body coil because of lack of perfect homogeneity of the main magnetic field from one side of the body to the other, aliasing of one side of the body to the other results in the superimposition of signals of different phases that add and cancel?
   a. Moire fringes.
   b. Zipper artifact.
   c. starry sky artifact.
   d. Zebra stripes.

5. The artifact appears as a focal dot of increased signal in the center of an image. Is it caused by a constant offset of the DC voltage in the receiver?
   a. Central point artifact.
   b. Zipper artifact.
   c. Zebra stripes
   d. Starry sky artifact.

6. A nonuniform, washed-out appearance to an image occurring when the signal received by the scanner from the patient is too intense to be accurately digitized by the analog-to-digital converter?
   a. RadioFrequency(RF) overflow artifact
   b. Zipper artifact
   c. Zebra stripe artifact
   d. Starry sky artifact

7. Losing signal intensity in one part of the image, leading to dark shading in this portion of the image caused by an uneven excitation of nuclei within the field; due to RF pulses applied at flip angles other than 90 and 180 degrees or by an abnormal loading of coil or coupling of coils at a point (as with a large patient who touches one side of the coil?
   a. Shading artifact.
   b. Zipper artifact.
   c. Starry sky artifact
   d. Aliasing artifact

8. An artifact in MRI occurs when the field of view (FOV) is smaller than the body part being imaged?
   a. Wrap-around or Aliasing artifact?
   b. Shading artifact.
   c. Zipper artifact.
   d. Starry sky artifact.

9. An artifact encountered in Magnetic Resonance imaging is a nonuniform distribution of image noise, typically affecting the center part of the image (being more distant from the surface coils) than the superficial tissues?
   a. Starry sky artifact
   b. Zipper Artifact
   c. Cross-excitation artifact
   d. Aliasing artifact

10. The artifact caused by reducing signal because of slice selection, there is the excitation of the adjacent slices, and if the adjoining portion is imaged during the same TR or imaging without a gap?
    a. Cross-excitation artifact.
    b. Zipper artifact
    c. Starry sky artifact
    d. Aliasing artifact

11. The effect in which the lesions appear more significant than their actual size is called?
    a. Blooming effect.
    b. Abtropung effect.
    c. Bystander effect.
    d. Zooming effect.

12. The artifact that occurs in Magnetic Resonance Imaging in the frequency-encoding direction because of spatial misregistration of fat and water molecules?
    a. Chemical shift artifact.
    b. Zipper artifact.
    c. Aliasing artifact.
    d. Starry sky artifact.

13. The artifact obtained during Magnetic Resonance Imaging (MRI) with above 3Tesla units in patients with ascites or Pregnant patients, when abdominal diameters exceed RF wavelength leading to darkening or shading at the center of the image due to constructive or destructive interference patterns?
    a. Dielectric effect artifact.
    b. Aliasing artifact.
    c. zipper artifact.
    d. starry sky artifact.

14. The artifact that appears as lines in the MR image parallel to abrupt and intense changes in the object at this location, such as the skull-brain and cerebrospinal fluid - spinal cord interface?
    a. Gibb's artifact.
    b. Aliasing artifact.
    c. Zipper artifact.
    d. Dielectric effect artifact.

15. The Magnetic resonance imaging caused by tightly bound collagenous areas results in short T2 time, resulting in lack of signal?
    a. Magic angle artifact.
    b. Gibbs artifact.
    c. Aliasing artifact.
    d. Dielectric effect artifact.

16. The artifact in Magnetic Resonance Imaging due to data in the k-space array missing or set to zero during scanning. The abrupt change from signal to no signal results in artifacts in the images showing alternating bands of shading and darkness, often in an oblique direction?
    a. Zero-fill artifact.
    b. Gibbs artifact.
    c. Dielectric effect artifact.
    d. Aliasing artifact.

17. The abstract concept in Magnetic Resonance Imaging that refers to data matrix containing raw MRI data?
    a. K-space
    b. L-space
    c. M-space
    d. N-space.

18. The reconstruction algorithm used in Magnetic Resonance Imaging?
    a. Fourier transform
    b. Feldkamp algorithm.
    c. Sinogram algorithm
    d. Inverse algorithm

19. The 3.0 Tesla Nuclear Magnetic Resonance Imaging system compared to the 1.5 Tesla Nuclear Magnetic Resonance imaging system?
    a. Higher Noise
    b. Low Spatial resolution.
    c. Low Specific absorption Rate.
    d. Low signal-to-noise ratio.

20. The Nuclear Magnetic resonance imaging system with the magnetic field of 3.0 Tesla is preferred to diagnose?
    a. Internal derangement of the articular disc.
    b. Condylar movement.
    c. Ankylosis.
    d. Subluxation.

Answers

1. a. Zipper artifact.
2. a. Corduray artifact.
3. a. Zebra stripes.
4. a. Moire fringes.
5. a. Central point artifact.
6. a. Radiofrequency (RF) overflow artifact.
7. a. Shading artifact.
8. a. Wrap around or Aliasing artifact.
9. a. Starry-sky Artifact.
10. a. Cross-excitation Artifact.
11. a. Blooming effect.
12. a. Chemical shift artifact.
13. a. Dielectric effect artifact.
14. a. Gibbs artifact.
15. a. Magic angle artifact.
16. a. Zero-fill artifact.
17. a. K-Space.
18. a. Fourier transform.
19. a. Higher noise.
20. a. Internal derangement of the articular disc.

Chapter 60

Positron Emission Tomography (PET)

Questions

1. The scintillation cameras used in Positron Emission Tomography are called?
    a. Anger cameras
    b. Dual cameras
    c. Auto cameras
    d. Semi-auto cameras

2. The scintillator used in photomultiplier tubes in Positron Emission Tomography is?
    a. Thallium activated sodium iodide.
    b. Terbium activated sodium iodide.
    c. Ruthenium activated sodium iodide.
    d. Cadmium activated sodium iodide.

3. One of the best and most used scintillators in time-of-flight positron emission tomography (TOF-PET) with one of the highest time photon densities is?
    a. Cerium-doped lutetium Oxyorthosilicate $Lu(2-x)\ YxSiO_5$ (LYSO: Ce).
    b. MDP
    c. Caesium iodide
    d. Bismuth Germinate

4. The technetium 99m administered intravenously in Positron Emission Tomography scan emits?
    a. Alpha radiation
    b. Beta radiation
    c. Gamma radiation
    d. Delta radiation.

5. Anger cameras in Positron Emission Tomography was invented in 1950s by?
    a. Hal Anger
    b. Paul ehrlich
    c. Lauterber
    d. Godfrey Hounsfield.

6. The Gamma camera is found combined with a CT scanner?
   a. Single Positron Emission Computed Tomography.
   b. Cone-beam Computed Tomography.
   c. Positron Emission Tomography.
   d. orthopantomography.

7. The imaging modality that differentiates condylar hyperplasia from condylar hypertrophy?
   a. Positron Emission Tomography (PET)
   b. Computed Tomography (CT)
   c. Magnetic Resonance Imaging (MRI)
   d. Ultrasonography.

8. Which of the following element used as scintillation detectors is highly hygroscopic in PET scan machines?
   a. Sodium Iodide (NaI)
   b. Bismuth Germanate (Bi4 Ge3 012)
   c. Barium Fluoride (Ba F2).
   d. Cadmium Tungstate. (CdWO4).

9. The main disadvantage of Sodium Iodide Crystals is?
   a. Low detection efficiency of Gamma rays with energies above 200 Kev.
   b. Low detection efficiency of Gamma rays with energies above 100 KeV.
   c. Low detection efficiency of Gamma rays with energies above 50 KeV.
   d. Low detection efficiency of Gamma rays with energies above 40 KeV.

10. The contrast medium used for Positron Emission Tomography scan is?
    a. 18 F-Fluorodeoxyglucose.
    b. Technetium pertechnetate.
    c. Radioactive chromium.
    d. Radon.

11. The valuable imaging modality for imaging, restaging, monitoring in Lymphomas?
    a. PET (Positron Emission Tomography).
    b. CT (Computed Tomography).
    c. Orthopantomography (OPG).
    d. Intraoral Periapical radiographs.

Answers

1. a. Anger cameras.
2. a. Thallium activated sodium iodide.
3. a. cerium-doped lutetium Oxyorthosilicate Lu(2−x) $YxSiO_5$ (LYSO: Ce).
4. c. Gamma radiation.
5. a. Hal Anger.
6. c. Positron Emission Tomography.
7. a. Positron Emission Tomography (PET).
8. a. Sodium Iodide.
9. a. Low detection efficiency of Gamma rays with energies above 200 Kev.
10. a. 18 F-Fluorodeoxyglucose.
11. a. PET(Positron Emission Tomography).

Chapter 61

SPECT

Questions

1. The imaging of choice for diagnosing Alzhiemer's disease, dementia, or Parkinsonism?
   a. CT.
   b. MRI.
   c. PET.
   d. SPECT.

2. The two-radiopharmaceutical used in the diagnosis of Brain perfusion studies is?
   a. 133- Xenon.
   b. ^{123}I -IMP (123I-Isopropyliodoamphetamine)
   c. Helium.
   d. ^{99m} Tc – Hexamethyl Propylene Amine Oxime (HMPAO) and ^{99m}Tc – Ethyl Cysteinate Dimer (ECD).

3. The specialized scan that helps to diagnose Pulmonary embolism is?
   a. Ventilation / Perfusion scan (V/Q).
   b. CT.
   c. MRI.
   d. CBCT.

4. A vasodilatory challenge is stated in the evaluation of cerebrovascular reserve in TIA, completed stroke, carotid artery stenosis or occlusion, and vascular anomalies; evaluation of the results of carotid surgery; preoperative assessment of the need for selective carotid shunting during carotid endarterectomy; and evaluation of cerebrovascular reserve before and after cerebrovascular surgery or stent placement; and to aid in distinguishing vascular from neuronal causes of dementia?
   a. Acetazolamide.
   b. Nicorandil.
   c. Cyclosporine.
   d. Nifedipine.

5. The stationary detectors do not overlap?
   a. U-SPECT -I
   b. U-SPECT-II
   c. X-SPECT.
   d. Nano-SPECT.

6. The Phenomenon in which projections can overlap called Multiplexing is possible?
   a. X-SPECT.
   b. U-SPECT-I.
   c. U-SPECT-II.
   d. U-SPECT-III.

7. The SPECT system that has stationary detectors?
   a. USEPECT-I.
   b. U-SPECT-II.
   c. X-SPECT.
   d. Nano- SPECT.

8. The collimator in U-SPECT II Consists?
   a. 0.35 mm UHR 75 Pinholes Focused Mouse collimator.
   b. 0.9 mm UHR 9 Pinholes/Plates.
   c. 1.2 mm; 5 Pinholes.
   d. 1.5 mm; 4 Pinholes.

9. The highest resolution is seen among the following SPECT Systems?
   a. U-SPECT-II.
   b. Nano SPECT.
   c. X-SPECT.
   d. U-SPECT-I.

10. The increased uptake occurs at the site of cerebral infarct in the brain called?
    a. Luxury Perfusion Phenomenon.
    b. Perfusion Phenomenon.
    c. Diffusion Phenomenon.
    d. Ventilation Phenomenon.

11. SPECT help in identifying unilateral epileptic focus during ictal and post-ictal stages by subtraction technology using?
    a. Feldkamp algorithm.
    b. Herm BRASS software.
    c. Davies algorithm.
    d. Kemp algorithm.

Answers

1. d. SPECT
2. d. ^{99m} Tc – Hexamethyl Propylene Amine Oxime (HMPAO) and ^{99m}Tc – Ethyl Cysteinate Dimer (ECD).
3. a. Ventilation / Perfusion scan (V/Q).
4. a. Acetazolamide.
5. b. U-SPECT –II.
6. a. X-SPECT.
7. b. USEPECT-II.
8. a. 0.35 mm UHR 75 Pinholes Focused Mouse collimator.
9. a. USPECT-II.
10. a. Luxury Perfusion Phenomenon.
11. b. Herm BRASS software.

Chapter 62

Cone Beam Computed Tomography (CBCT) Imaging

Questions

1. The multiple sequential planar projection images obtained, as the x-ray source and detector move through an arc of 180 to 360 degrees, are called?
   a. Raw images.
   b. Cone beam images.
   c. Inverse images.
   d. Back projection images.

2. The method of obtaining data from two or more separate scans and superimposing the overlapping regions of the CBCT data volumes using corresponding fiducial reference landmarks is called?
   a. Bioimage registration.
   b. Scout registration.
   c. Bite registration.
   d. Heterogeneous registration.

3. The fusion of adjacent image volumes to create a more extensive volumetric set in the horizontal or vertical dimension is called?
   a. Stitching.
   b. Destiching.
   c. Switching.
   d. Deswitching.

4. The CBCT units with these detectors are bulkier?
   a. Image intensifier/Charged coupled Device (II/CCD).
   b. Complementary metal oxide sensor.
   c. Charge injection Device.
   d. Photostimulable Phosphor plates.

5. The CBCT units with Image Intensifier/charge-coupled device (II/ CCD) combination have the following volume?
   a. Spherical volume.
   b. Circular volume.
   c. Cone-shaped volume.
   d. Square-shaped volume.

6. The CBCT units with a Flat panel detector have the following shape of the volume?
   a. Cylindrical volumes.
   b. Circular volumes.
   c. Cone-shaped volume.
   d. Rectangular volumes.

7. The flat panel detectors in CBCT machines comprise the following?
   a. Cesium iodide scintillator to a transistor made of amorphous silicon.
   b. Barium iodide scintillator to a transistor made of amorphous silicon.
   c. Potassium iodide scintillator to a transistor made of amorphous silicon.
   d. Fluoroiodide scintillator to a transistor made of amorphous silicon.

8. What is the individual volume elements produced in CBCT formatting the volumetric data set?
   a. Pixels.
   b. Voxels.
   c. Axis.
   d. Scout.

9. The CBCT produces Voxel resolution equal in all three dimensions called?
   a. Anisotropic.
   b. Isotropic.
   c. Heterotropic.
   d. Ectopic.

10. The following parameter determines the number of shades of grey available and helps to display differences in attenuation?
    a. Pixel depth.
    b. Voxel depth.
    c. Isotropic depth.
    d. Bit depth.

11. The CBCT units can record Greyscale values?
    a. 11 bits or higher.
    b. 12 bits or higher.
    c. 13 bits or higher.
    d. 14 bits or higher.

12. A 12-bit CBCT detector provides a display?
    a. 4056 shades of gray.
    b. 4076 shades of gray.
    c. 4086 shades of gray.
    d. 4096 shades of gray.

13. A 16-bit CBCT detector provides a display?
    a. 65,526 shades of gray.
    b. 65,536 shades of gray.
    c. 65,546 shades of gray.
    d. 65,556 shades of gray.

14. The processing of basis images into a volumetric data set is called?
    a. Primary reconstruction.
    b. Secondary reconstruction.
    c. Tertiary reconstruction.
    d. Primitive reconstruction.

15. A composite image developed from acquired multiple planar Projection images is called?
    a. Sinogram.
    b. Pictogram.
    c. Histogram.
    d. Pixel.

16. The process of generation of sinogram in a CBCT is called?
    a. Radon transformation.
    b. Bizarre transformation.
    c. Pixel.
    d. Inverse radon transformation.

17. The final image reconstructed from sinogram with a filtered back-projection algorithm for volumetric data acquired by CBCT imaging is called?
    a. Inverse Radon Transformation.
    b. Radon transformation.
    c. Pixel.
    d. Voxel.

18. These items are instructed to be removed by the patient before subjecting them to CBCT, EXCEPT?
    a. Eyeglasses.
    b. Earrings.
    c. Nose Piercings.
    d. Complete removable acrylic Prosthesis.

19. The fraction of a pixel's area capable of collecting light is called?
    a. Fill factor.
    b. K-factor.
    c. H-factor.
    d. P-factor.

20. The reduction in patient dose is usually associated with a reduction in (Field of Volume) FOV, which results in a dose reduction?
    a. 5-10%
    b. 10-15%
    c. 25-66%
    d. 35-76%

Answers

1. a. Raw images.
2. a. Bioimage registration.
3. a. Stitching.
4. a. Image intensifier/ charged coupled Device (II/CCD).
5. a. Spherical volume.
6. a. Cylindrical Volumes.
7. a. Cesium iodide scintillator to a transistor made of amorphous silicon.
8. b. Voxels.
9. b. Isotropic.
10. d. Bit depth.
11. b. 12 Bits or Higher.
12. d. 4096 Shades of Grey.
13. b. 65,536 shades of Grey.
14. a. Primary reconstruction.
15. a. Sinogram.
16. a. Radon Transformation.
17. a. Inverse Radon Transformation.
18. d. Complete Removable Acrylic Prostheses.
19. b. K-Factor.
20. c. 25- 66%.

Chapter 63

CBCT - Volume Preparation

Questions

1. The four technical stages that provide an efficient and consistent methodological approach to optimize CBCT image display before image interpretation EXCEPT?
   a. Reorient the data.
   b. Optimize the data.
   c. View the data.
   d. Reformat the data.

2. The reviewing of each series dynamically by scrolling consecutively through an orthogonal image stack is called?
   a. Paging mode.
   b. Magnification mode.
   c. Display mode.
   d. View mode.

3. The basic format options in CBCT include all the following EXCEPT?
   a. Multiplanar reformation.
   b. Volumetric rendering.
   c. Ray sum.
   d. Display mode.

4. The volumetric data set can be sectioned non orthogonally to provide nonaxial two-dimensional planar images called?
   a. Multiplanar reformation.
   b. Maximum intensity projection.
   c. Display mode.
   d. Scout image.

5. The slice thickness of orthogonal images can be thickened by increasing the number of adjacent voxels included in the display, which creates an image that represents a specific volume of the patient. What is it called?
   a. Ray sum.
   b. Volumetric rendering.
   c. Display mode.
   d. Field of volume.

6. Which of the following allows visualization of volumetric data by the selective display of voxels within a data set?
   a. Volumetric rendering.
   b. Ray sum.
   c. Field of volume.
   d. Field of interest.

7. A complex process requiring selecting the intensity or density of the grayscale level of the voxels to be displayed within an entire data set?
   a. Volumetric rendering.
   b. Field of volume.
   c. Ray sum.
   d. Segmentation.

8. The phenomenon of volumetric rendering is optimal for the following?
   a. Relationship of an inferior alveolar canal to the mandibular third molar.
   b. Field of volume.
   c. Field of interest.
   d. Display.

9. A more straightforward process in which an arbitrary threshold of voxel intensities is selected and all gray values above or below are eliminated?
   a. Maximum intensity Projections.
   b. Field of interest.
   c. Field of volume.
   d. Display.

10. What is the stent made with radiographic markers inserted during the scan, which precisely locates the proposed implants or teeth, is called?
    a. Diagnostic stent.
    b. Surface stent.
    c. Locator stent.
    d. Depth stent.

11. The main indication of CBCT over conventional radiographs is that?
    a. To locate the exact cause for periapical pathology, whether external or internal resorption or invasive cervical resorption.
    b. Locate periosteal blood vessels.
    c. Locate sinus opening.
    d. Locate fine cracks in the enamel.

12. The process of integrating two imaging data sets such as extraoral photographic data set or optical intraoral impression data sets in CBCT is called?
    a. Image fusion.
    b. Ray sum.
    c. Segmentation.
    d. Stitching.

13. The techniques that translate software-derived virtual surgical plans developed from virtual simulations to the surgical environment are called?
    a. Image-guided surgery.
    b. Image-guided regeneration.
    c. Image-guided embracement.
    d. Image-guided drilling.

14. A broad term used to describe a group of related processes and techniques used to fabricate physical scale models directly from three-dimensional computer-assisted design data is called?
    a. Rapid Prototyping.
    b. Image-guided surgery.
    c. Image-guided regeneration.
    d. Ray sum.

15. The purpose of Rapid prototyping in the maxillofacial region is to create a life-size, dimensionally accurate model of an anatomical structure called?
    a. Bio models.
    b. Ray sum.
    c. Segmentation.
    d. Stitching.

Answers

1. d. Reformat the Data.
2. a. Paging Mode.
3. d. Display Mode.
4. a. Multiplanar reformation.
5. a. Ray sum.
6. a. Volumetric Rendering.
7. d. Segmentation.
8. a. Relationship of an inferior alveolar canal to the Mandibular Third Molar.
9. a. Maximum Intensity Projection.
10. a. Diagnostic stent.
11. a. To locate the exact cause for periapical pathology, whether external or internal resorption or invasive cervical resorption.
12. a. Image Fusion.
13. a. Image-Guided Surgery.
14. a. Rapid Prototyping.
15. a. Bio models.

Chapter 64

CBCT Artifacts

Questions

1. What is any distortion or error in the image unrelated to the subject being studied is called?
   a. Noise.
   b. Artifact.
   c. Resolution.
   d. Magnification.

2. CBCT has more artifacts than MDCT because of all the following, EXCEPT?
   a. Higher energy spectra were used.
   b. Cone beam geometry.
   c. Higher noise level.
   d. Scatter.

3. The following are the cone-beam-related artifacts in CBCT, EXCEPT?
   a. Scatter.
   b. Cone -beam effect.
   c. Partial volume averaging.
   d. Magnification.

4. The following inherent artifact occurs in CBCT because diffracted x-ray photons from their original path after attenuation were captured by the detector, resulting in overall image degradation are called?
   a. Scatter.
   b. Partial volume averaging.
   c. Cone -beam effect.
   d. Magnification.

5. The artifact that results when the selected voxel size of the scan is larger than the size of the object being imaged is called?
   a. Partial volume averaging.
   b. Scatter.
   c. Cone -beam effect.
   d. Magnification.

6. The following bone architecture is more prone for Partial volume averaging artifact?
   a. Mandible.
   b. Maxilla.
   c. Temporal bone.
   d. Alveolar bone.

7. The following artifact results during CBCT scan, especially in the peripheral portion of scan volume, because of the divergence of the x-ray beam in a horizontal plane, the structures on the top and bottom of the image are exposed only when the x-ray source is on the opposite side of the patient?
   a. Cone -beam effect.
   b. Scatter.
   c. Magnification.
   d. Distortion.

8. The reduced data sample that leads to misregistration, sharp edges, and noisier images can cause the following in the obtained image?
   a. Fine striations.
   b. Distortion.
   c. Graininess.
   d. Noise.

9. The poor calibration or imperfections in the scanner detector of CBCT results?
   a. Circular artifacts.
   b. Cylindrical artifacts.
   c. Spherical artifacts.
   d. Octagonal artifacts.

10. The phenomenon in which passing a cone-shaped beam through an object results in the preferential absorption of low energy photons in preference to high energy photons?
    a. Beam hardening.
    b. Circular artifact.
    c. Motion artifact.
    d. Cone-beam effect.

11. The artifact in which streak and dark bands create the following artifact when present between two dense objects?
    a. Beam hardening.
    b. Circular artifact.
    c. Extinction artifact.
    d. Motion artifact.

12. The patient's movement during the CBCT Scan can cause misregistration of data, which appear as double contours in the reconstructed image is called?
    a. Motion artifacts.
    b. Beam hardening.
    c. Cone- beam effect.
    d. Extinction artifact.

13. CBCT can produce images of submillimeter voxel resolution in all orthogonal planes of about?
    a. 0.005-0.1010 mm.
    b. 0.0076-0.125 mm.
    c. 0.007-0.2020 mm.
    d. 0.076-0.226 mm.

14. The substantial dose reduction by CBCT compared to MDCT is?
    a. 430-1160μSv.
    b. 330-1060μSv.
    c. 220-1160μSv.
    d. 110-1060μSv.

15. What is the scattered beam to Primary radiation ratios in CBCT imaging?
    a. 0.2-2
    b. 0.3-2
    c. 0.4-2
    d. 0.5-2

16. What are the statistical variations in the homogeneity of the incident x-ray beam that can cause image noise in CBCT is called?
    a. Quantum mottle.
    b. Scatter.
    c. Missing artifacts.
    d. Motion artifacts.

17. The inherent degradations of the detector system related to the x-ray absorption efficiency of energy at the detector are called?
    a. Electronic noise.
    b. Scatter.
    c. Missing artifacts.
    d. Motion artifacts.

18. What effect is caused by the increased divergence of the x-ray beam over the area detector called?
    a. Heel effect.
    b. Photoelectric effect.
    c. Bohr effect.
    d. Abscopal effect.

19. The heel effect that causes nonuniformity or considerable variation of the incident cone-shaped x-ray beam on the patient and greater signal to noise?
    a. Greater on the anode side.
    b. Greater on the cathode side.
    c. Equal on both cathode and anode sides.
    d. Less on the cathode and anode side.

20. What are the Flat panel detector-based artifacts that affect linearity or response to cone beam x-ray radiation?
    a. Saturation.
    b. Dark current.
    c. Bad pixel.
    d. Pixel -pixel gain non-variation.

Answers

1. b. Artifacts.
2. a. Higher energy spectra used.
3. d. Magnification.
4. a. Scatter.
5. a. Partial volume averaging.
6. c. Temporal Bone.
7. a. Cone Beam effect.
8. a. Fine striations.
9. a. Circular artifacts.
10. a. Beam Hardening.
11. c. Extinction artifact.
12. a. Motion artifacts.
13. b. 0.076 – 0.125 mm.
14. a. 430 – 1160 μSv.
15. c. 0.4 -2
16. a. Quantum Mottle.
17. a. Electronic noise.
18. a. Heel effect.
19. b. Greater on Cathode side.
20. d. Pixel-Pixel Gain Non-variation.

Chapter 65

Dental Implant Imaging

Questions

1. The percentage of mandibular periapical radiographs do not demonstrate the mandibular canal is?
   a. 15%
   b. 25%
   c. 35%
   d. 45%

2. Lateral cephalometric imaging provides a known magnification for the midline structures?
   a. 7-12%
   b. 8-12%
   c. 9-12%
   d. 10-12%

3. The horizontal image magnification with panoramic radiographs ranges from?
   a. 0.7-2.2 times.
   b. 0.5-2.0 times
   c. 0.6-2.3 times.
   d. 0.4-2.4 times.

4. The choice of radiographic technique helps in the placement of some implants near midline for overdentures?
   a. Lateral cephalometric radiograph.
   b. Orthopantamograph.
   c. Zimmers projection.
   d. Transcranial projection.

5. The radiograph used as a screening for preliminary assessment of crestal alveolar bone, cortical boundaries of the mandibular canal, maxillary sinus?
   a. Orthopantamograph.
   b. Lateral Cephalometric radiograph.
   c. Transorbital projection.
   d. Transcranial projection.

6. Is the voxel size required for implant imaging irrespective of field of volume (FOV)?
   a. 0.3 to 0.4 mm.
   b. 0.2 to 0.3 mm.
   c. to 0.2 mm.
   d. 0.4 to 0.5 mm.

7. Magnetic resonance imaging is contraindicated in patients with?
   a. Ferromagnetic implants.
   b. Diamagnetic implants.
   c. Paramagnetic implants.
   d. Titanium implants.

8. The minimum amount of residual bone surrounding the implant must be?
   a. 1 to 1.5mm.
   b. 2 to 3 mm.
   c. 3 to 4 mm.
   d. 4 to 5 mm.

9. The amount of bone between the implant and adjacent structures such as the mandibular canal and Nasal fossa?
   a. 2 to 3 mm.
   b. 1 to 2 mm.
   c. 3 to 4 mm.
   d. 4 to 5 mm.

10. The image obtained by the following in which the actual size of the jaw can be calibrated without magnification?
    a. CBCT imaging software.
    b. Panoramic radiograph.
    c. Lateral cephalometric radiograph.
    d. Transcranial radiograph.

11. The following type of implants do not produce an axial scatter artifact?
    a. Root form implants.
    b. Basal implants.
    c. Ferromagnetic implants.
    d. Mini implants.

12. The angulation must be within the following degrees of the long axis of the fixture to open the threads on the image on most threaded fixtures?
    a. 6 degrees.
    b. 7 degrees.
    c. 8 degrees.
    d. 9 degrees.

13. The angulation of more than following degrees can completely overlap the threads?
    a. 12 Degrees.
    b. 13 Degrees.
    c. 14 Degrees.
    d. 15 Degrees.

14. The radiographic sign which indicates failure of osseointegration is?
    a. Saucerization.
    b. Coronal migration of alveolar bone.
    c. Increased radiodensity of alveolar bone.
    d. An increased trabecular pattern of alveolar bone.

15. Which radiographic appearance indicates the poor stress distribution from implant abutment prosthesis?
    a. Widening of Periodontal Ligament space.
    b. Crestal alveolar bone loss.
    c. The radiolucent area following the outline of an implant.
    d. Apical migration of alveolar bone

16. The radiograph indicating the improper non-axial loading from improper angulation of the implant is shown in the radiograph?
    a. Apical migration on one side of the implant.
    b. The radiolucent area following the outline of an implant.
    c. Crestal alveolar bone loss.
    d. Saucerization.

Answers

1. b. 25%.
2. a. 7-12 %
3. a. 0.7-2.2 times.
4. a. Lateral Cephalometric radiograph.
5. a. Orthopantamography.
6. a. 0.3-0.4 mm.
7. a. Ferromagnetic implants.
8. a. 1-1.5 mm.
9. b. 1- 2mm.
10. a. CBCT imaging software.
11. a. Root form implants.
12. d. 9 degrees.
13. b. 13 degrees.
14. a. Saucerization.
15. a. Widening of Periodontal Ligament Space.
16. A. Apical migration on one side of the implant.

Chapter 66

Nanoparticles in Biomedical Imaging

Questions

1. The following nanoparticles are used for the detection of Nucleic acids?
   a. Gold.
   b. Silver.
   c. Platinum.
   d. Palladium.

2. The following nanoparticles are used as contrast agents in computed tomography to detect Head and Neck cancers?
   a. Gold nanoparticles.
   b. Silver nanoparticles.
   c. Platinum nanoparticles.
   d. Rubidium nanoparticles.

3. The fluorescent semiconductor nanocrystals have advantages in medical imaging when paired with the potential for in vivo targeting of specific neoplastic cells, DNA after conjugation with specific bioactive moieties, hence useful for fluorescence imaging?
   a. Quantum Dots.
   b. Gold Spheres.
   c. Gold rods.
   d. Palladium rods.

4. The nanoparticle used to target integrin-rich tumor cells?
   a. Gold spheres.
   b. Quantum dots.
   c. Ultrasmall Iron oxide nanoparticles (USPION).
   d. Gold rods.

5. Carbon Nanotubes were discovered?
   a. Paatero.
   b. Thompson.
   c. Black.
   d. Iiijima.

6. The following property of single-walled nanotubes is helpful as contrast agents?
   a. Near Infra-Red Fluorescence. (NIR)
   b. Near Ultra Violet Fluorescence. (NUVF)
   c. Hyper resonance.
   d. Hypo resonance.

7. The capacity of Fluorescence-induced Isothiocyanate -labeled single-walled nanotubes to penetrate the cells was studied using?
   a. Epifluorescence and confocal microscopy.
   b. Stereoscopy.
   c. Colposcopy.
   d. Dermascopy.

8. The following nanoparticles are explored as gene or drug delivery systems?
   a. Polyamidoamine (PAMAM) and Polypropyleneimine (PPI).
   b. Polyamidoimine (PAMIM) and Polyimine (PI).
   c. Polyimidoimine (PIMIM) and Polyamine (PA).
   d. Polypropyleneimine (PPLIM) and Polyamidoamine (PAA).

9. The nanoparticles used as contrast agents for assessment of tumor angiogenesis?
   a. PerfluorocarbonNanoparticles (PFCNP)
   b. Polyamidoamine (PAMAM)
   c. Polypropyleneimine (PPI)
   d. Polyamide (PA).

10. The following nanoparticles can help identify and locate the disease and provide information about the treatment response?
    a. Theranostic nanoparticles.
    b. Polyamide.
    c. Gold spheres.
    d. Quantum dots.

11. The material used for coating various types of nanoparticles, thus producing particles with multiple functions and identifying various diseases?
    a. Chitosan.
    b. Polyamide.
    c. Gold spheres.
    d. Quantum dots.

12. The amalgamation of three types of Liposomes, namely conventional, PEGylated and ligand targeted types, is called?
    a. Theranostic Liposome.
    b. polyamidoamine (PAMAM).
    c. Quantum dots.
    d. Gold spheres.

13. The following are the mechanism for the controlled release of drugs for nanocarriers, EXCEPT?
    a. Diffusion.
    b. Chemical reactions.
    c. Stimuli were sensitive.
    d. Reduction.

Answers

1. a. Gold.
2. a. Gold Nanoparticles.
3. a. Quantum dots.
4. c. Ultrasmall Iron oxide nanoparticles (USPION).
5. d. Ijiima.
6. d. Hyporesonance.
7. a. Epifluorescence and confocal microscopy.
8. a. Polyamidoamine (PAMAM) and Polypropyleneimine (PPI).
9. a. Perfluorocarbon Nanoparticles (PFCNP).
10. a. Theranostic nanoparticles.
11. a. Chitosan.
12. a. Theranostic Liposome.
13. d. Reduction.

Chapter 67

Radioprotectors and Radiosensitisers

Questions

1. The Radiosensitizer that helps inhibit tumor growth by enhanced sensitivity through Target regenerating Gene (REGIII)?
   a. Resveratrol.
   b. Quercetin.
   c. Genistein.
   d. Kaempferol.

2. The Radiosensitizer that helps in targeting squamous cell carcinoma cells by targeting antioxidant enzyme thioredoxin reductase-1 (TxnRd1)?
   a. Resveratrol.
   b. Genistein.
   c. Kaempferol.
   d. Curcumin.

3. A significant compound of soy that plays a vital role in tumor suppression by activating the AKT gene and mediating G2 M arrest?
   a. Quercetin.
   b. Genistein.
   c. Kaempferol.
   d. Curcumin.

4. The Polysaccharide Radiosensitizers highly effective on Human Melanoma cells?
   a. Quercetin.
   b. Fucoidans.
   c. Huaier.
   d. Ginseng.

5. A polyphenolic compound used as a radiosensitizer in Nasopharyngeal carcinoma enhances radiosensitivity in Nasopharyngeal carcinoma by inhibiting NF (Nuclear Factor) – kappa pathway?
   a. Caffeic acid Phenylethyl Ester.
   b. Huaier.
   c. Ginseng.
   d. Quercetin.

6. A radiosensitizer that is less toxic and effective in sensitizing hypoxic tumor cells?
   a. Nimorazole.
   b. Metronidazole.
   c. Tinidazole.
   d. Fluconazole.

7. A novel radioprotective drug that protects human lymphoblastoid cells reducing radiation-induced DNA strand breaks?
   a. Tetracycline.
   b. Metronidazole.
   c. Amifostine.
   d. Glutathione.

8. A novel camptothecin derivative radiosensitizer that exerts its cytotoxic effect by targeting DNA Topoisomerase I?
   a. Irinotecan.
   b. Amifostine.
   c. Glutathione.
   d. Cysteine.

9. A Texaphyrin-based radiosensitizer?
   a. Motexafin Gadolinium.
   b. Amifostine.
   c. Carbogen.
   d. Glutathione.

10. A radiosensitizing non-nucleoside analog acts by inhibiting ribonucleotide reductase, a critical enzyme that prevents the transformation of ribonucleotides to deoxyribonucleotides?
    a. Hydroxyurea.
    b. Amifostine.
    c. Carbogen.
    d. Irinotecan.

Answers

1. a. Resveratrol
2. d. Curcumin.
3. b. Genestein.
4. b. Fucoidans.
5. a. Caffeic acid Phenylethyl ester.
6. a. Nimorazole.
7. a. Tetracycline.
8. a. Irinotecan.
9. a. Motexafin Gadolinium.
10. a. Hydroxyurea.

Chapter 68

Radiological Signs and Appearances

Questions

1. Bow sign is a feature of which carcinoma?
   a. Nasopharyngeal carcinoma.
   b. Verrucous carcinoma.
   c. Squamous cell carcinoma.
   d. Basal cell carcinoma.

2. Tail sign is a feature?
   a. Plunging ranula.
   b. Sublingual space infection.
   c. Submandibular space infection.
   d. Submental space infection.

3. Rice grain calcifications are seen?
   a. Cysticercosis.
   b. Myiasis.
   c. Trypanosomiasis.
   d. Hydatid cyst.

4. Copper-beaten appearance of the skull?
   a. Hydrocephalus.
   b. Craniosynostosis.
   c. Meningioma.
   d. Glioma.

5. Lacunar skull is seen?
   a. Myelomeningocele.
   b. Hydrocephalus.
   c. Thalassemia.
   d. Glioma.

6. The appearance of Bull horn occurs?
   a. SAPHO syndrome.
   b. LEOPARD syndrome.
   c. Noonan syndrome.
   d. Turcot's syndrome.

7. Black sign is a radiological feature?
   a. Coccidiomycosis.
   b. Blastomycosis.
   c. Mucormycosis.
   d. Histoplasmosis.

8. Lincoln beard sign is a feature of scintigraphy examination?
   a. Fibrous dysplasia.
   b. Paget's disease.
   c. Osteopetrosis.
   d. Osteoporosis.

9. Codman's triangle is a radiological feature seen?
   a. Osteosarcoma.
   b. Malignant melanoma.
   c. Hemangiopericytoma.
   d. Paget's disease.

10. Driven snow appearance is a characteristic radiological feature seen in the following cyst?
    a. Calcifying epithelial odontogenic Tumour.
    b. Radicular cyst.
    c. Ameloblastoma.
    d. Dentigerous cyst.

11. Donut appearance is seen in the following Hamartoma?
    a. Dens Evaginatus.
    b. Dens invaginatus.
    c. Odontome.
    d. Mandibular Torus.

12. Toadstool appearance of the condyle?
    a. Juvenile arthritis.
    b. Osteoarthritis.
    c. Psoriatic arthritis.
    d. Gonococcal arthritis.

13. The "Sausage link appearance "under sialography is seen?
    a. Sialodochitis.
    b. Sialadenitis.
    c. Salivary gland tumors.
    d. Sialosis.

14. What is the sialographic appearance of fruit-laden "cherry blossom" seen?
    a. Sialadenitis.
    b. Sialosis.
    c. Sjogren syndrome.
    d. Sialodochitis.

15. A Tram Track sign can be seen?
    a. Sturge Weber syndrome.
    b. Cowden syndrome.
    c. Rutherford syndrome.
    d. Apert syndrome.

16. The imaginary lines used in Waters radiograph to assess fracture of middle third of the facial skeleton?
    a. Mc Grigor and Campbell Lines.
    b. Innominate lines.
    c. Lines of Trochanter.
    d. Curve of Spee.

17. What are the imaginary lines used in evaluating maxillofacial fractures in the occipitomental radiograph?
    a. Mc Grigor and Campbell Lines.
    b. Innominate Lines.
    c. Dolan Lines.
    d. Lines of Trochanter.

18. Which of the following has a trap door sign as a feature?
    a. Zygomatic arch fracture.
    b. Nasal bone fracture.
    c. Blow out fracture of the orbital floor.
    d. Mandibular Fracture.

19. Wimberger ring sign, a circular calcification around the epiphyseal center of ossification, is seen?
    a. Vitamin A deficiency.
    b. Scurvy.
    c. Rickets.
    d. Osteoporosis.

20. The serpent sign, which can be seen on ultrasound, CT, or MRI, is a feature?
    a. Dermoid cyst.
    b. Thyroglossal cyst.
    c. Hydatid cyst.
    d. Nasopalatine cyst.

21. What is the Panda Sign a feature?
    a. Fracture of the mandible.
    b. Fracture of Maxilla.
    c. Fracture of the Base of the skull.
    d. Fracture of the zygoma.

22. The Comb sign is a feature?
    a. Crohn's Disease.
    b. Hepatitis.
    c. Pancreatitis.
    d. Maxillofacial Trauma.

23. Carman's meniscus sign is a feature?
    a. Peptic ulcer.
    b. Gastric ulcer.
    c. Duodenal ulcer.
    d. Ulcer of the small intestine.

24. The "Pelvic brim sign "is a radiological sign seen?
    a. Paget's disease.
    b. Osteoporosis.
    c. Osteopetrosis.
    d. Fibrous Dysplasia.

25. Sandwich sign is a feature of MRI?
    a. Primary Pleural Lymphoma.
    b. Nonhodgkins Lymphoma.
    c. Multiple Myeloma.
    d. Osteosarcoma.

26. The volcano sign is seen in MRI in the following brain tumor?
    a. Meningioma.
    b. Glioma.
    c. Meningocele.
    d. Pyocele.

27. Is the rind sign near the proximal portions of the long bone femur characteristic?
    a. Fibrous dysplasia.
    b. Osteoporosis.
    c. Osteosarcoma.
    d. Paget's disease.

28. Open ring sign is a feature?
    a. Stroke.
    b. Parkinsonism.
    c. Multiple sclerosis.
    d. Hemiplegia.

29. Comma sign in CT, seen?
    a. Subdural Haematomas.
    b. Extradural Haematomas.
    c. Fracture Maxilla.
    d. Fracture of Mandible.

30. Donut sign in the Bone scan is seen?
    a. Simple Bone cyst.
    b. Fibrous dysplasia.
    c. Paget's disease.
    d. Osteopetrosis.

31. Troisier sign is a feature?
    a. Gastric carcinoma.
    b. Basal cell carcinoma.
    c. Malignant melanoma.
    d. Verrucous carcinoma.

32. Garrington sign, is seen?
    a. Osteosarcoma.
    b. Chondrosarcoma.
    c. Synovial sarcoma.
    d. Meningioma.

33. String sign of Kantor is seen?
    a. Crohn's Disease.
    b. Gastric carcinoma.
    c. Pyrolic carcinoma.
    d. Carcinoma of Duodenum.

34. Panda sign in Gallium -67 citrate scan is a feature?
    a. Sarcoidosis.
    b. Tuberculosis.
    c. Emphysema.
    d. Pleural effusion.

35. What is the Bare orbit sign seen due to the destruction of an innominate line?
    a. Neurofibromatosis Type I.
    b. Osteoma.
    c. Chondroma.
    d. Paget's disease.

36. Double skull sign is a feature of CT?
    a. Late Calcified Cephalohematomas.
    b. Early calcified cephalohematomas.
    c. Subdural Hematomas.
    d. Extradural Hematomas.

37. Lyre sign, the splaying of the external and internal carotid artery is a feature?
    a. Adamantinoma.
    b. Carotid Body tumor.
    c. Aortic aneurysms.
    d. Fallot's tetralogy.

38. Turtleback sign is a feature?
    a. Schistosomiasis.
    b. Trypanosomiasis.
    c. Filariasis.
    d. Cysticercosis.

39. Step ladder pattern in Intraoral periapical radiograph is a feature?
    a. Iron deficiency anemia.
    b. Megaloblastic anemia.
    c. Aplastic anemia.
    d. Cooley's anemia.

40. Hair on end appearance on Lateral skull radiograph is a feature?
    a. Thalassemia.
    b. Megaloblastic anemia.
    c. Aplastic anemia.
    d. Iron deficiency anemia.

41. Y sign is a feature of Lipoma?
    a. Face.
    b. Neck.
    c. Epidural space.
    d. Wrist.

42. The spade phalanx sign is a characteristic feature of the appearance of spade-shaped meta phalangeal bones in hand wrist radiographs?
    a. Acromegaly.
    b. Cretinism.
    c. Cushing's Disease.
    d. Addison's disease.

43. Concentric ring sign on MRI is a feature?
    a. Subacute Hematoma.
    b. Late Hematoma.
    c. Fracture of Maxilla.
    d. Fracture of Mandible.

44. Is a Snowman sign, Figure of 8, or Dumb Bell configuration an MRI feature seen?
    a. Pituitary Macroadenomas.
    b. Meningiomas.
    c. Gliomas.
    d. Malignant melanomas.

45. The following reveals a cord sign in non-contrast-enhanced CT?
    a. Dural Venous sinus Thrombosis.
    b. Thrombophlebitis.
    c. Vascular stenosis.
    d. Aneurysm of the cerebellar artery.

46. Cumbo sign is a feature?
    a. Hydatid cyst.
    b. Neurocysticercosis.
    c. Schistosomiasis.
    d. Trypanosomiasis.

47. Teardrop sign, due to the herniation of orbital fat with or without inferior rectus muscle occurs?
    a. Inferior orbital wall fracture.
    b. Apex of orbit fracture.
    c. Lateral orbital wall fracture.
    d. Medial orbital wall fracture.

48. Cluster of Black Pearls sign is a contrast-enhanced CT scan feature that helps differentiate lymphadenopathy from the following from other causes like Tuberculosis, Adenocarcinoma?
    a. Sarcoidosis.
    b. Aspergillosis.
    c. Mucormycosis.
    d. Histoplasmosis.

49. Polka dot sign is a feature?
    a. Haemangioma of Alveolar bone.
    b. Vertebral intraosseous Haemangiomas.
    c. Haemangioma of Femur.
    d. Haemangioma of Neck.

50. Light Bulb sign is a feature?
    a. Pituitary Macroadenomas.
    b. Phaeochromocytoma.
    c. Insulinoma.
    d. Cushing's Disease.

Answers

1. a. Nasopharyngeal carcinoma.
2. a. Plunging ranula.
3. a. Cysticercosis.
4. a. Hydrocephalus.
5. a. Myelomeningocele.
6. a. SAPHO Syndrome.
7. c. Mucormycosis.
8. b. Paget's disease.
9. a. Osteosarcoma.
10. a. Calcifying Epithelial Odontogenic Tumour.
11. c. Odontome.
12. a. Juvenile arthritis.
13. a. Sialodochitis.
14. c. Sjogren syndrome.
15. a. Sturge Weber syndrome.
16. a. Mc Grigor and Campbell Lines.
17. c. Dolan Lines.
18. c. Blow out fracture of orbital Floor.
19. b. Scurvy.
20. c. Hydatid cyst.
21. c. Fracture of Base of the skull.
22. a. Crohn's Disease.
23. b. Gastric Ulcer.
24. a. Paget's Disease.
25. a. Primary Pleural Lymphoma.
26. a. Meningioma.
27. a. Fibrous dysplasia.
28. c. Multiple sclerosis.
29. a. Subdural Haematoma.
30. a. Simple Bone cyst.
31. a. Gastric carcinoma.
32. a. Osteosarcoma.
33. a. Crohn's Disease.
34. a. Sarcoidosis.
35. a. Neurofibromatosis Type I.
36. b. Early calcified Cephalohematomas.
37. b. Carotid Body Tumour.

38. a. Schistosomiasis.
39. a. Iron deficiency anemia.
40. a. Thalassemia.
41. c. Epidural space.
42. a. Acromegaly.
43. a. Subacute Haematoma.
44. a. Pituitary Macroadenomas.
45. a. Dural Venous sinus thrombosis.
46. a. Hydatid cyst.
47. a. Inferior orbital wall fracture.
48. a. Sarcoidosis.
49. b. Vertebral intraosseous Haemangiomas.
50. b. Phaeochromocytoma.

Chapter 69

Artificial Intelligence

Questions

1. The study of algorithms that give machines the ability to reason and perform functions such as problem-solving, object and word recognition, inference of world states, and decision-making?
   a. Intelligent Quotient.
   b. Artificial Intelligence.
   c. Normalization.
   d. Linearization.

2. Which of the following is not a technique used for Artificial intelligence?
   a. Fuzzy Logic.
   b. Neural Networks.
   c. Bayesian Method.
   d. Regression Model.

3. The Kalman Filter, a linear-quadratic algorithm that uses measurements observed over time, including statistical noises, provides a joint probability distribution over variables for each time frame using the following technique in Artificial intelligence?
   a. Bayesian Method.
   b. Neural Network.
   c. Fuzzy Logic.
   d. Linear Model.

4. The framework in which different machine learning algorithms work to achieve a particular task such as data classification, image recognition is called?
   a. Neural Network.
   b. Normalization.
   c. Quantification.
   d. Fuzzy Logic.

5. The main limitation of Artificial intelligence is that?
   a. Cannot determine a causal relationship.
   b. Cannot able to recognize Patterns.
   c. Not susceptible to Bias.
   d. An algorithm provides why a Prediction was made.

6. A form of machine learning in which multi-layered (deep) neural networks (NNs) are trained to learn features of complex data structures (e.g., image data or language)?
   a. Fuzzy Logic.
   b. Machine Learning.
   c. Deep Learning.
   d. Bayesian method.

7. The representation of intrinsic statistical patterns and structures in data allows predilections for unseen data?
   a. Deep Learning.
   b. Machine Learning.
   c. Linear model.
   d. Bias.

8. The first neural network was developed?
   a. Minsky and Dean Edmunds.
   b. Lotfe Zaidi.
   c. Caudell.
   d. Mizel.

9. The term "Fuzzy Logic "was coined?
   a. Lotfe Zaedi.
   b. Mizel.
   c. Caudell.
   d. Dean Edmunds.

10. The term "Augmented reality" is coined?
    a. Lofte Zaidi.
    b. Edmunds.
    c. Caudell and Mizel.
    d. Black.

Answers

1. b. Artificial intelligence.
2. d. Regression Model.
3. a. Bayesian method.
4. d. Fuzzy Logic.
5. a. Cannot determine a causal relationship.
6. b. Machine learning.
7. a. Deep Learning.
8. a. Minsky and Dean Edmunds.
9. a. Lofti Zaedi.
10. c. Caudell and Mizel.

Chapter 70

Quality Assurance in Radiology

Questions

1. The term used to describe the administrative and Technical efforts made to identify and correct equipment Problems before they have become so severe as to affect the diagnostic quality of the radiographs being produced?
   a. Quality Assurance.
   b. Retake Log.
   c. Reference film.
   d. Legal aspects.

2. The instrument used for measuring density, the degree of darkness of exposed and processed radiographic film?
   a. Densitometer.
   b. Spin top test.
   c. Penny test.
   d. Thermoluminescent dosimeter.

3. The following is used to check the timer in an x-ray machine?
   a. Spinning -top test.
   b. Dosimeter.
   c. Densitometer.
   d. Penny test.

4. The milli-Ampere (mA) of the dental x-ray machine can be checked?
   a. Voltmeter.
   b. Densitometer.
   c. Ammeter.
   d. Kilovoltmeter.

5. The test of placing several aluminum sheets of various thicknesses between the position indicating device and Dosimeter is to test?
   a. Milli-Ampere (m A)
   b. Half Value Layer (HVL)
   c. Density.
   d. Safelight illumination.

6. A 6-inch plastic cylinder with paired slots in a wafer of lead that are closer and closer together at one end and the other is open is called?
   a. Focal Spot checker.
   b. Penny test.
   c. Densitometer.
   d. Step wedge test.

7. The help of a coin can test the following?
   a. Safelight.
   b. Half value layer.
   c. Collimator.
   d. Timer.

8. A spinning top is used to check the?
   a. Density.
   b. Collimator.
   c. Timer.
   d. Filter.

9. The device that measures the radiation output is?
   a. Pocket Dosimeter.
   b. Densitometer.
   c. Focal spot checker.
   d. Filter.

10. The device used in conjunction with the densitometer to check the processing quality?
   a. Sensitometer.
   b. Dosimeter.
   c. Ammeter.
   d. Focal spot checker.

11. While testing the collimator, the diameter of the exposed area must not be greater than?
   a. 5 cm.
   b. 6 cm.
   c. 7 cm.
   d. 8 cm.

12. A device that exposes the film to a calibrated light pattern is?
   a. Sensitometer.
   b. Densitometer.
   c. Step wedge.
   d. Spinning top.

Answers

1. a. Quality Assurance.
2. a. Densitometer.
3. a. Spinning- top test.
4. c. Ammeter.
5. b. Half Value Layer (HVL).
6. a. Focal Spot checker.
7. a. Safelight.
8. c. Timer.
9. a. Pocket Dosimeter.
10. a. Sensitometer.
11. c. 7 cm.
12. a. Sensitometer.

Chapter 71

Infection Control in Radiology

Questions

1. The infection control procedures designed to protect workers from exposure to diseases spread by blood and certain body fluids, including saliva, is called?
   a. Standard Precautions.
   b. Careful Precautions.
   c. Safe Precautions.
   d. Good Precautions.

2. The items that do not come in contact with oral mucous membrane such as a dental chair, headrest, lead apron, control panel in the x-ray machine, thyroid collar is called?
   a. Noncritical items.
   b. Critical items.
   c. Semi-critical items.
   d. Semi-noncritical items.

3. An effective barrier for dental x-ray consoles is?
   a. Plastic wrap.
   b. Iodine disinfectant.
   c. Soap solution.
   d. Cetrimide solution.

4. The plastic wraps are conveniently stored?
   a. Butcher's Paper dispenser mounted on a wall.
   b. Table.
   c. Near Dental chair.
   d. Near Headrest.

5. Does the American Dental Association recommend that any chemical disinfectant be an Environmental Protection Agency (EPA) -registered Hospital Disinfectant?
   a. High activity.
   b. Low-intermediate activity
   c. Very High activity.
   d. Very Low activity.

6. The items that do not penetrate soft tissue or bone but contact the oral mucous membrane?
   a. Critical items.
   b. Semi-critical items.
   c. Noncritical items.
   d. Crucial items.

7. Immersion of the exposed film in the following disinfectant solution is effective?
   a. 5.25% sodium hypochlorite for 30 secs.
   b. 0.2% chlorhexidine solution for 30 secs.
   c. 0.1% sodium bicarbonate for 30 secs.
   d. 0.1% saline for 30 secs.

8. The disinfectant solution used must be at least?
   a. Tuberculocidal.
   b. Tuberculostatic.
   c. Bactericidal.
   d. Bacteriostatic.

9. What are the disinfectants suggested for Panoramic bite blocks, chin rest, and cephalostat ear post?
   a. Detergent-iodine disinfectant.
   b. Glutaraldehyde.
   c. Sodium hypochlorite.
   d. Benzalkonium chloride.

10. What is the recommended immersion time for disinfection in 5.25% sodium hypochlorite solution?
    a. 20 Seconds.
    b. 30 Seconds.
    c. 40 Seconds.
    d. 50 Seconds.

Answers

1. a. Standard Precautions.
2. a. Noncritical items.
3. a. Plastic wrap.
4. a. Butcher's Paper Dispenser mounted on a wall.
5. b. Low- intermediate activity.
6. b. Semi- Critical items.
7. a. 5.25% Sodium Hypochlorite for 30 secs.
8. a. Tuberculocidal.
9. a. Detergent-iodine disinfectant.
10. b. 30 seconds.

Chapter 72

Normal Radiological Anatomical Landmarks in Maxilla

Questions

1. A thin radiolucent line extending between the long axis of the roots of Maxillary central incisors?
   a. Median Palatal suture.
   b. Incisive fossa.
   c. Nasal cavity.
   d. Lateral fossa.

2. The diffuse radiolucent area between the maxillary lateral incisor and maxillary canine is?
   a. Lateral Fossa.
   b. Median Palatine suture.
   c. Nasal fossa.
   d. Incisive fossa.

3. The radiopaque projection within the nasal cavity is called?
   a. Inferior Nasal Concha.
   b. Middle Nasal concha.
   c. Superior Nasal concha.
   d. Lateral Nasal concha.

4. The intersection forms the inverted "Y"?
   a. Anterior border of Maxillary sinus and Lateral wall of Nasal Fossa.
   b. The posterior border of Maxillary sinus and Medial Wall of Nasal Fossa.
   c. The superior border of the Maxillary sinus and Anterior wall of the Nasal Fossa.
   d. The inferior border of the Maxillary sinus and Posterior wall of the Nasal Fossa.

5. The radiopaque landmark that appears as a radiopaque bulge distal to the Maxillary third molar area?
   a. Maxillary sinus.
   b. Maxillary tuberosity.
   c. The antrum of Highmore.
   d. Zygomatic Process of Maxilla.

6. Is the hook-like projection seen posterior to Maxillary tuberosity in an intraoral periapical radiograph of the Maxillary Posterior region?
   a. Hamulus.
   b. Tuberosity.
   c. Nasal septum.
   d. The floor of the Maxillary sinus.

7. The J or U-shaped radioopaque projection superimposed on the periapical root region of Maxillary molars is?
   a. Zygomatic Process of Maxilla.
   b. Maxillary Tuberosity.
   c. Nasal septum.
   d. Hamulus.

8. The radiopaque partitions seen within the Maxillary sinus?
   a. Bony septum.
   b. Inferior Nasal concha.
   c. Middle Nasal concha.
   d. Superior Nasal concha.

9. The clinical significance of Median Palatine suture or Intermaxillary suture is that?
   a. It aids in Rapid Maxillary Expansion using Fixed Functional appliances.
   b. It prevents fracture of the Hard Palate.
   c. It helps in the distribution of occlusal forces.
   d. It retards the Growth of the Hard Palate.

10. A "V" Shaped radiopaque area at the intersection of the floor of the nasal cavity and nasal septum in periapical radiograph of the maxillary anterior region?
    a. Nasal fossa.
    b. Anterior Nasal spine.
    c. Hamulus.
    d. Nasal septum.

11. A triangular radiopaque projection that occurs in a Maxillary posterior intraoral radiographs superimposed over or inferior to the Maxillary Tuberosity region is?
    a. Coronoid Process of Mandible.
    b. Condylar Process of Mandible.
    c. Zygomatic Process of Maxilla.
    d. Hamular Process of Sphenoid.

12. The following is the predominant shape of the Greater Palatine canal in Axial Cone Beam computed Tomography section?
    a. Oval.
    b. Hourglass.
    c. Circular.
    d. Square.

13. The following is the predominant shape of the Greater Palatine canal in Sagittal Cone Beam computed Tomography section?
    a. Oval.
    b. Square.
    c. Hourglass.
    d. Comma.

14. The anatomical structure that carries anterior superior alveolar nerve and is often overlooked in cone-beam computed Tomography can?
    a. Canalis sinuous.
    b. Nasopalatine canal.
    c. Mid Palatine suture.
    d. Anterior Nasal Spine.

15. The canalis sinuosis is more predominant in the following anatomical region?
    a. Anterior Maxilla; Between Maxillary central and Lateral incisor.
    b. Anterior Mandible; Between Maxillary Lateral incisor and Maxillary canine.
    c. Posterior Maxilla; Between Maxillary Premolars and Maxillary Molars.
    d. Posterior Mandible; Between Mandible Premolars and Mandibular Molars.

16. The additional radiolucent canal behind the maxilla's incisive foramen that transmits the nasopalatine nerve?
    a. Foramina of Scarpa.
    b. Foramen rotendum.
    c. Foramen spinosum.
    d. Foramen ovale.

Answers

1. a. Median Palatal Suture.
2. a. Lateral Fossa.
3. a. Inferior Nasal concha.
4. a. Anterior border of Maxillary sinus and Lateral wall of Nasal Fossa.
5. b. Maxillary Tuberosity.
6. a. Hamulus.
7. a. Zygomatic Process of Maxilla.
8. a. Bony septum.
9. a. It aids in Rapid Maxillary Expansion using Fixed Functional appliances.
10. b. Anterior Nasal Spine.
11. a. Coronoid Process of the mandible.
12. a. Oval.
13. c. Hourglass.
14. a. Canalis sinuosis.
15. b. Anterior Mandible; Between Maxillary Lateral incisor and Maxillary canine.
16. a. Foramina of Scarpa.

Chapter 73

Normal Radiological Anatomical Landmarks in Mandible

Questions

1. A ring-shaped radiopaque structure is seen in the periapical radiographs of the mandibular anterior teeth region?
   a. Genial Tubercles.
   b. Lingual Foramen.
   c. Mental Foramen.
   d. Mandibular Foramen.

2. A small radiolucent dot-like structure within the ring-like radiopacity with the periapical region of the mandibular anterior region is?
   a. Mental foramen.
   b. Mandibular foramen.
   c. Lingual foramen.
   d. Foramen ovale.

3. The vertical tube-like passages that carry blood vessels and appear as vertical radiolucent lines with the long axis of the mandibular anterior teeth region and steep radiopaque tube-like courses with the long axis of the mandibular posterior region are?
   a. Nutrient canals.
   b. Mandibular foramen.
   c. Mental foramen.
   d. Lingual Foramen.

4. A small radiolucent area in the apical region of mandibular Premolars is?
   a. Lingual Foramen.
   b. Mandibular Foramen.
   c. Mental Foramen.
   d. Nutrient canals.

5. A dense radiopaque band-like structure that gets superimposed over the image of the roots of mandibular posterior teeth?
   a. Mylohyoid ridge.
   b. External oblique ridge.
   c. Mental ridge.
   d. Internal oblique ridge.

6. A radiopaque band extending downward and forward from the anterior border of the ramus of the mandible and typically ends in the Mandibular third molar region is?
   a. External oblique ridge.
   b. Mental ridge.
   c. Mylohyoid ridge.
   d. Internal oblique ridge.

7. The average height of the alveolar crest appears?
   a. 1.5 to 2mm below Cementoenamel Junction.
   b. 1 to 1.5 mm below cementoenamel Junction.
   c. 0.5 to 1 mm below cementoenamel Junction.
   d. 2 to 2.5 mm below cementoenamel Junction.

8. The Periodontal Ligament space measures?
   a. 0.1 mm
   b. 0.2 mm
   c. 0.3 mm
   d. 0.4 mm

9. The cyst-like radiolucency below the level of the mandibular canal and above the lower border in Infront of the angle of the mandible caused by steepened submandibular gland fossa?
   a. Stafne defect.
   b. Fenestration.
   c. Dehiscence.
   d. Residual cyst.

10. The cyst-like defect caused by steepened sublingual fossa and occur in the mandibular anterior region?
   a. Submandibular fossa.
   b. Stafne defect.
   c. Anterior lingual defect.
   d. Submental fossa.

Answers

1. a. Genial Tubercles.
2. c. Lingual foramen.
3. a. Nutrient canals.
4. c. Mental foramen.
5. a. Mylohyoid ridge.
6. a. External oblique ridge.
7. a. 1.5 to 2mm below Cementoenamel Junction.
8. b. 0.2 mm.
9. a. Stafne defect.
10. c. Anterior lingual defect.

Chapter 74

Principles of Radiographic Interpretation

Questions

1. Who stated that radiographic appearances are governed by anatomic and physiologic changes in the presence of disease processes?
   a. Black.
   b. Laskin.
   c. Worth.
   d. Okeson.

2. The point of origin of lesion that assists in indicating the tissue types that compose this abnormality is called?
   a. Epicenter.
   b. Foci.
   c. Focal spot.
   d. Focal trough.

3. The fusiform expansion of the inferior alveolar canal indicates a lesion of which origin?
   a. Neural.
   b. Odontogenic.
   c. Vascular.
   d. Cartilaginous.

4. The trabecular pattern in Fibrous dysplasia is usually?
   a. More significant in number, Shorter, randomly oriented.
   b. Lesser in number, Longer, non-randomly oriented.
   c. More significant in number, Larger, aligned in response to stress.
   d. Lesser in number, Larger, not aligned in response to stress.

5. Which of the following lesion push the tooth apically EXCEPT?
   a. Follicular cyst.
   b. Odontomas.
   c. Lymphomas.
   d. Circumferential Dentigerous cyst.

6. The lesion that has a curved, coarse septa due to cystic formation within the lesion remodels the trapped bone into curved shapes?
   a. Dentigerous cyst.
   b. Odontogenic Myxoma.
   c. Ameloblastoma.
   d. Adenomatoid odontogenic tumor.

7. The location of the epicenter above the following anatomical landmark suggests its odontogenic origin of any lesion?
   a. Inferior alveolar canal.
   b. Nasal cavity.
   c. Orbit.
   d. Zygoma.

8. The following internal septations are seen in Giant cell granuloma?
   a. wispy or granular septations.
   b. Straight septations.
   c. Curved, coarse septa.
   d. Unilocular straight internal septa.

9. The space-occupying lesion slowly creates space by displacing the teeth?
   a. Cyst.
   b. Abscess.
   c. Phlegmon.
   d. Granuloma.

10. The following is a multifocal lesion?
    a. Keratocystic odontogenic tumor.
    b. Dentoalveolar Abscess.
    c. Cellulitis.
    d. Periapical granuloma.

Answers

1. c. Worth.
2. a. Epicenter.
3. a. Neural.
4. a Greater in number, Shorter, randomly oriented.
5. c. Lymphomas.
6. c. Ameloblastomas.
7. a. Inferior alveolar canal.
8. a. Wispy or granular septations.
9. a. Cyst.
10. a. Keratocystic odontogenic tumor.

Chapter 75

Radiographic Film Holders

Questions

1. The holder used in Bisecting angle technique is?
   a. RINN-SNAP-A-RAY.
   b. RINN-X-C-P.
   c. Paper Loop receptor holder.
   d. BAI Bite Block.

2. The holder used in Paralleling or Long cone technique is?
   a. RINN -SNAP-A-RAY.
   b. RINN-X-C-P.
   c. Paper Loop receptor holder.
   d. BAI Bite Block.

3. The holder used for the Bitewing radiographic technique?
   a. RINN -SNAP-A-RAY.
   b. RINN X-C-P
   c. Paper Loop receptor holder.
   d. BAI Bite Block.

4. A specialized radiographic film holder that allows files to be in place when subject to radiograph to make a radiographic image?
   a. RINN SNAP-A-RAY.
   b. RINN X-C-P
   c. Paper Loop receptor holder.
   d. EndoRay.

5. The following film holder is used for accurate positioning of the sensor for distortion-free images?
   a. RINN SNAP-A-RAY.
   b. RINN X-C-P
   c. EEZEE Grip.
   d. Endoray.

6. The radiographic film holder for the tooth with files in the root canal?
   a. Paper Loop receptor holder.
   b. RINN SNAP-A-RAY.
   c. RINN X-C-P.
   d. Endoray.

7. The radiographic film holder has three detachable parts Guiding frame, an L-shaped metal rod frame, a plastic tab for holding the film?
   a. RINN X-C-P.
   b. RINN SNAP-A-RAY.
   c. Paper Loop receptor holder.
   d. BAI bite block.

8. The radiographic film holder used for holding Photostimulable Phosphor Plates?
   a. RINN X-C-P.
   b. RINN SNAP-A-RAY.
   c. BAI bite block.
   d. Paper Loop receptor holder.

9. The chances of film bend do not occur in the following radiographic film holder?
   a. RINN SNAP-A-RAY.
   b. Paper loop receptor holder.
   c. RINN X-C-P.
   d. EEZEE Grip.

10. The following instrument can be used as a film holder for the mandibular third molar?
    a. Haemostat.
    b. EEZEE grip.
    c. Paper Loop receptor holder.
    d. BAI Bite block.

Answers

1. a. RINN-SNAP-A-RAY
2. b. RINN X-C-P.
3. c. Paper Loop receptor holder.
4. d. Endoray.
5. c. EEZEE Grip.
6. d. Endoray.
7. a. RINNX-C-P.
8. c. BAI bite block.
9. c. RINN X-C-P.
10. a. Haemostat.

Chapter 76

Radiotherapy Techniques

Questions

1. A form of radiotherapy placed sealed radioactive sources directly in or next to the tumor to be treated directly or with catheters?
   a. Teletherapy.
   b. Brachytherapy.
   c. Intensity-modulated radiotherapy.
   d. Stereotactic radiotherapy.

2. The implantation of radioactive sources close to the tumor is called?
   a. Plesiotherapy.
   b. Stereotactic radiotherapy.
   c. Intensity Modulated radiotherapy.
   d. Proton therapy.

3. The most common advantage of Brachytherapy is?
   a. Requires selection of additional Target Tumour volume
   b. Rapid dose falls off of adjacent areas of the Target volume of Tumour.
   c. Toxicity in proximity to critical organs near Tumour.
   d. Invasive.

4. The most common form of Brachytherapy used to treat head and neck cancers for early T1 lesions involving Lip, Buccal Mucosa, Tongue, Floor of the mouth?
   a. Interstitial.
   b. Surface mold.
   c. Bead technique.
   d. Intraluminal.

5. The technique of Brachytherapy used to cover upper, and superior surface underdose on the dorsum of the tongue is?
   a. Bead technique.
   b. Mesh technique.
   c. Pellet technique.
   d. Cone technique.

6. The material used for Nasopharyngeal Brachytherapy is?
   a. Rotterdam's Nasopharyngeal Brachytherapy applicator.
   b. Amsterdam's Nasopharyngeal Brachytherapy applicator.
   c. Hamsterdam's Nasopharyngeal Brachytherapy applicator.
   d. Collendam's Nasopharyngeal Brachytherapy applicator.

7. The Brachytherapy used to treat Head and Neck cancers in the Hard Palate, External ear?
   a. Interstitial
   b. Intraluminal.
   c. Surface mold.
   d. Bead technique.

8. The Brachytherapy used for the treatment of Nasopharyngeal carcinoma is?
   a. Interstitial.
   b. Intraluminal.
   c. Bead.
   d. Surface mold.

9. The pulsed dose rate Brachytherapy is used to treat?
   a. Lip carcinoma.
   b. Carcinoma of alveolus.
   c. Carcinoma of Maxilla.
   d. Carcinoma of the condyle.

10. The radioisotope of choice used for irradiation by Brachytherapy for recurrent Carcinoma of Head and Neck region after surgical resection is?
    a. Cesium-131 seeds.
    b. Iodine 131.
    c. Cobalt wires.
    d. Radon seeds.

11. The following is used during interstitial brachytherapy treatment of hypopharyngeal carcinoma to create a space between clinical target volume and organs at risk?
    a. Polymethylmethacrylate spacer.
    b. Polyethylene glycol hydrogel spacer or hyaluronate spacer gel.
    c. Titanium mesh.
    d. Vitallium mesh.

12. The shape of the collimators used in Intensity-modulated radiotherapy is?
    a. Peacock shaped.
    b. Circular shaped.
    c. Square shaped.
    d. Rectangle-shaped.

13. The radiotherapy technique used in the treatment of Hodgkin's Lymphoma?
    a. Mantle field.
    b. Doppler field.
    c. Magnetic field.
    d. Electro field.

14. What is the radiotherapy technique that aims to precisely position the patient to deliver a more accurate radiotherapy beam at the target tumor volume called?
    a. Intensity Guided Radiotherapy.
    b. Intensity Modulated Radiotherapy.
    c. Mantle field radiotherapy.
    d. Arc technique.

15. The Volumetric Modulated Arc therapy has an advantage over Intensity Modulated radiotherapy EXCEPT?
    a. Rapid treatment time.
    b. Decreased Radiation dosage to the target tumor.
    c. More sparing of adjacent healthy tissues.
    d. Decreased homogeneity of radiation dose.

16. A painless computed guided radiotherapy treatment procedure for treating idiopathic Trigeminal neuralgia is?
    a. Gamma Knife.
    b. Volumetric modulated arc therapy.
    c. Intensity Modulated Radiotherapy.
    d. Intensity Guided Radiotherapy.

17. The technique of delivering radiotherapy for tumors located in moving parts such as the lung, abdomen?
    a. Respiratory Gating Technique.
    b. Volumetric Modulated arc therapy.
    c. Intensity Modulated Radiotherapy.
    d. Intensity Guided Radiotherapy.

Answers

1. b. Brachytherapy.
2. a. Plesiotherapy.
3. b. Rapid dose falls off of adjacent areas of the Target volume of Tumour.
4. a. Interstitial Brachytherapy.
5. a. Bead technique.
6. a. Rotterdam's Nasopharyngeal Brachytherapy applicator.
7. c. Surface mold.
8. b. Intraluminal.
9. a. Lip carcinoma.
10. a. Caesium-131 seeds.
11. b. Polyethylene glycol hydrogel spacer or hyaluronate spacer gel.
12. a. Peacock shaped.
13. a. Mantle field.
14. a. Intensity Guided Radiotherapy.
15. d. Decreased homogeneity of radiation dose.
16. a. Gamma Knife.
17. a. Respiratory Gating Technique.

References

Oral Medicine

Chapter 1

Burket's oral medicine, 11th edition, In chapter: Red and white lesions of the oral cavity. Page: 77-106.

Chapter 2

Burket's oral medicine, 11th edition, In chapter: Red and white lesions of the oral cavity. Page: 77-106.

Chapter 3

Burket, oral medicine, 11th edition, Chapter 4: Red and white lesions of the oral mucosa, Page: 77-106.

Chapter 4

Burket's oral medicine. 11th edition, Chapter 5: Pigmented lesions of the oral cavity. Page: 107-128.

Chapter 5

Khailany R. A., Safdar M., Ozaslan M. Genomic characterization of a novel SARS-CoV-2. *Gene Rep*. 2020,19 doi: 10.1016/j.genrep.2020.100682.

Samudrala PK, Kumar P, Choudhary K, et al. Virology, pathogenesis, diagnosis and in-line treatment of COVID-19. *Eur J Pharmacol*. 2020,883:173375. doi:10.1016/j.ejphar.2020.173375.

Walls A. C., Park Y.-J., Tortorici M. A., Wall A., McGuire A.T., Veesler D. Structure, function, and Antigenicity of the SARS-CoV-2 Spike glycoprotein. *Cell*. 2020, 181:281–292. doi: 10.1016/j.cell.2020.02.058. e6.

Yüce, M., Filiztekin, E., & Özkaya, K. G. (2021). COVID-19 diagnosis -A review of current methods. *Biosensors & bioelectronics*, *172*, 112752. https://doi.org/10.1016/j.bios.2020.112752.

Chapter 6

Burket's oral medicine. 11th edition, Chapter 3: Ulcerative, vesicular and Bullous lesions. Page no:41-76.

Chapter 7

Burket's oral medicine. 11th edition, Chapter 3: Ulcerative, vesicular and Bullous lesions. Page no:41-76.

Tavakolpour, S., Soori, T., Noormohammadpour, P., Balighi, K., Mahmoudi, H., & Daneshpazhooh, M. (2017). Rituximab administration in a patient with pemphigus vulgaris following reactivation of occult hepatitis B virus infection. *Dermatology online journal*, *23*(6), 13030/qt8927s9kt.

Chapter 8

Koch, A., & Mizrahi, V. (2018). Mycobacterium tuberculosis. *Trends in microbiology*, *26*(6), 555–556. https://doi.org/10.1016/j.tim.2018.02.012.

Singh Bakshi S. (2017). A lumpy jaw. Mandíbula abultada. *Medicina clinica*, *149*(1), e5. https://doi.org/10.1016/j.medcli.2016.09.035.

Chapter 9

Whitley RJ. Herpesviruses. In: Baron S, editor. *Medical Microbiology*. 4th edition. Galveston (TX): University of Texas Medical Branch at Galveston, 1996. Chapter 68. Available from: https://www.ncbi.nlm.nih.gov/ books/NBK8157/.

Chapter 10

Adesiyun OA, Adeoye PO, Ofoegbu CK, Fadeyi A, Oyinloye OI, Atobatele MO. Candida esophagitis: Feathery appearance as a new sign on barium esophagogram. *West Afr J Radiol* 2015,22: 110-2.

Arvanitis M, Mylonakis E. Diagnosis of invasive aspergillosis: recent developments and ongoing challenges. *Eur J Clin Invest*. 2015,45(6):646-652. doi:10.1888888888888888111/eci.12448.

Clancy, C. J., & Nguyen, M. H. (2018). Diagnosing Invasive Candidiasis. *Journal of clinical microbiology*, *56*(5), e01909-17. https://doi.org/10.1128/ JCM.01909-17.

Clark NM, Grim SA, Lynch JP 3rd. Posaconazole: Use in the Prophylaxis and Treatment of Fungal Infections. *Semin Respir Crit Care Med.* 2015,36(5):767-785. doi:10.1055/s-0035-1562902.

Cornely OA, Arikan-Akdagli S, Dannaoui E, et al. ESCMID and ECMM joint clinical guidelines for the diagnosis and management of mucormycosis 2013. *Clin Microbiol Infect.* 2014,20 Suppl 3:5-26. doi:10.1111/1469-0691.12371.

Debi, U., Sharma, M., Singh, L., & Sinha, A. (2019). Barium esophagogram in various esophageal diseases: A pictorial essay. *The Indian journal of radiology & imaging*, *29*(2), 141–154. https://doi.org/10.4103/ijri. IJRI_465_18.

Farraia, M. V., Cavaleiro Rufo, J., Paciência, I., Mendes, F., Delgado, L., & Moreira, A. (2019). The electronic nose technology in clinical diagnosis: A systematic review. *Porto biomedical journal*, *4*(4), e42. https://doi.org/ 10.1097/j.pbj.0000000000000042.

Gomes, M. Z., Lewis, R. E., & Kontoyiannis, D. P. (2011). Mucormycosis caused by unusual mucormycetes, non-Rhizopus, -Mucor, and -Lichtheimia species. *Clinical microbiology reviews*, *24*(2), 411–445. https://doi.org/10. 1128/CMR.00056-10.

Heddergott C, Calvo AM, Latgé JP. The volatome of Aspergillus fumigatus. *Eukaryot Cell.* 2014,13(8):1014-1025. doi:10.1128/EC.00074-14.

Maziarz, E. K., & Perfect, J. R. (2016). Cryptococcosis. *Infectious disease clinics of North America*, *30*(1), 179–206. https://doi.org/10.1016/j.idc. 2015.10.006.

Nadkarni T, Goel A. Aspergilloma of the brain: an overview. *J Postgrad Med.* 2005, 51 Suppl 1:S37-S41.

Sullivan T, Meenakshi Rana, *The Reverse halo sign and Mucormycosis, Lancet, Infectious diseases* (2019).

Chapter 11

In *Oral Radiology, Principles and interpretation*, Stuart C. White, Michael. J. Pharoah, first south asia edition, In chapter: 27. Temporomandibular Joint abnormalities. Page 509.

Chapter 12

Jang DW, Comer BT, Lachanas VA, Kountakis SE. Aspirin sensitivity does not compromise quality-of-life outcomes in patients with Samter's triad. *Laryngoscope*. 2014 Jan,124(1):34-7. doi: 10.1002/lary.24220. Epub 2013 Jun 28. PMID: 23712910.

Chapter 13

Oral Radiology, Principles and interpretation, First south Asia edition, Stuart. C. White, Michael. J. Pharoah. In chapter 21: Cysts.

Chapter 14

Oral Radiology, Principles and interpretation, First south Asia edition, Stuart. C. White, Michael. J. Pharoah. In chapter 22: Benign Tumors.

Chapter 15

Oral Radiology, Principles and interpretation, First south Asia edition, Stuart. C. White, Michael. J. Pharoah. In chapter 23: Other Bone diseases. Page 402-425.

Chapter 16

Oral Radiology, Principles and interpretation, First south Asia edition, Stuart. C. White, Michael. J. Pharoah. In chapter 31: Other Bone diseases. Page 402-425.

Chapter 17

Narayanan LL, Vaishnavi C. Endodontic microbiology. *J Conserv Dent*. 2010 Oct, 13(4):233-9. doi: 10.4103/0972-0707.73386. PMID: 21217951, PMCID: PMC3010028.

Chapter 18

Mangold, A. R., Torgerson, R. R., & Rogers, R. S., 3rd (2016). Diseases of the tongue. *Clinics in dermatology*, *34*(4), 458–469. https://doi.org/10.1016/ j.clindermatol.2016.02.018.

Chapter 19

Gellrich, D., Bichler, M., Reichel, C. A., Schrötzlmair, F., & Zengel, P. (2020). Salivary Gland Disorders in Children and Adolescents: A 15-year Experience. *International archives of otorhinolaryngology*, *24*(1), e31–e37. https://doi.org/10.1055/s-0039-1697993.
Huzaifa, M., & Soni, A. (2021). Mucocele and Ranula. In *StatPearls*. StatPearls Publishing.

Chapter 20

Burket's oral medicine, 11 th edition, In chapter 22: Neuromuscular disorders. Page: 537-548.

Chapter 21

Burket's oral medicine, 11 th edition, In chapter 16: Haematological diseases. Page: 385-410.

Murray Longmore et al. *Oxford Handbook of clinical medicine*, oxford university press, 7th edition.

Chapter 22

Rumi, E., Baratè, C., Benevolo, G., Maffioli, M., Ricco, A., & Sant'Antonio, E. (2020). Myeloproliferative and lymphoproliferative disorders: State of the art. *Hematological oncology*, *38*(2), 121–128. https://doi.org/10.1002/ hon.2701.

Chapter 23

Meier, B., & Burton, J. H. (2017). Myeloproliferative Disorders. *Hematology/oncology clinics of North America*, *31*(6), 1029–1044. https://doi.org/10.1016/j.hoc.2017.08.007.

Chapter 24

Himes, C. P., Ganesh, R., Wight, E. C., Simha, V., & Liebow, M. (2020). Perioperative Evaluation and Management of Endocrine Disorders. *Mayo Clinic proceedings*, *95*(12), 2760–2774. https://doi.org/10.1016/j.mayocp. 2020.05.004.

Ruggeri, R. M., Giuffrida, G., & Campennì, A. (2018). Autoimmune endocrine diseases. *Minerva endocrinologica*, *43*(3), 305–322. https://doi.org/10. 23736/S0391-1977.17.02757-2.

Chapter 25

Ananthan, S., & Benoliel, R. (2020). Chronic orofacial pain. *Journal of neural transmission (Vienna, Austria: 1996)*, *127*(4), 575–588. https://doi.org/ 10.1007/s00702-020-02157-3.

Badel, T., Zadravec, D., Bašić Kes, V., Smoljan, M., Kocijan Lovko, S., Zavoreo, I., Krapac, L., & Anić Milošević, S. (2019). OROFACIAL PAIN - DIAGNOSTIC AND THERAPEUTIC CHALLENGES. *Acta clinica Croatica*, *58* (Suppl 1), 82–89. https://doi.org/ 10.20471/acc.2019.58.s1.12.

Christoforou J. (2018). Neuropathic Orofacial Pain. *Dental clinics of North America*, *62*(4), 565–584. https://doi.org/10.1016/j.cden.2018.05.005.

Crandall J. A. (2018). An Introduction to Orofacial Pain. *Dental clinics of North America*, *62*(4), 511–523. https://doi.org/10.1016/j.cden.2018.05.001.

Chapter 26

Liu, F., & Dang, Y. H. (2017). *Fa yi xue za zhi*, *33*(2), 175–180. https://doi.org/ 10.3969/j.issn.1004-5619.2017.02.015.

Prajapati, G., Sarode, S. C., Sarode, G. S., Shelke, P., Awan, K. H., & Patil, S. (2018). Role of forensic odontology in the identification of victims of major mass disasters across the world: A systematic review. *PloS one*, *13*(6), e0199791. https://doi.org/ 10.1371/journal.pone.0199791.

Chapter 27

In *Oral Radiology, Principles and interpretation*, Stuart C. White, Michael. J. Pharoah, first south Asia edition, In chapter: 34. Forensics. Page 646.

Chapter 28

Azarpazhooh, A., & Limeback, H. (2008). The application of ozone in dentistry: a systematic review of literature. *Journal of dentistry*, *36*(2), 104–116. https://doi.org/10.1016/j.jdent.2007.11.008.

Sen, S., & Sen, S. (2020). Ozone therapy a new vista in dentistry: integrated review. *Medical gas research*, *10*(4), 189–192. https://doi.org/10.4103/ 2045-9912.304226.

Silva, E., Prado, M. C., Soares, D. N., Hecksher, F., Martins, J., & Fidalgo, T. (2020). The effect of ozone therapy in root canal disinfection: a systematic review. *International endodontic journal*, *53*(3), 317–332. https://doi.org/10. 1111/iej.13229.

Tricarico, G., Rodrigues Orlandin, J., Rocchetti, V., Ambrosio, C. E., & Travagli, V. (2020). A critical evaluation of the use of ozone and its derivatives in dentistry. *European review for medical and pharmacological sciences*, *24*(17), 9071–9093. https://doi.org/10.26355/eurrev_202009_ 22854.

Tricarico, G., Rodrigues Orlandin, J., Rocchetti, V., Ambrosio, C. E., & Travagli, V. (2020). A critical evaluation of the use of ozone and its derivatives in dentistry. *European review for medical and pharmacological sciences*, *24*(17), 9071–9093. https://doi.org/10.26355/eurrev_202009_ 22854.

Chapter 29

Singal, A., & Arora, R. (2015). Nail as a window of systemic diseases. *Indian dermatology online journal*, *6*(2), 67–74. https://doi.org/10.4103/2229-5178.153002.

Chapter 30

Louppides S, Kakoullis L, Parpas G, et al. Upper eyelid oedema in a patient with pharyngitis/exudative tonsillitis and malaise: Hoagland sign in infectious mononucleosis *BMJ Case Reports CP* 2019,12:e233719.

Kulkarni AS, Birangane RS, Parkarwar PC, Kazi AZ. Clinical and radiological signs of importance for the oral physician and oral surgeon. *J Indian Acad Oral Med Radiol* 2019,31:257-62.

Chapter 31

Kaur, J., Jacobs, R., Huang, Y., Salvo, N., & Politis, C. (2018). Salivary biomarkers for oral cancer and pre-cancer screening: a review. *Clinical oral investigations*, *22*(2), 633–640. https://doi.org/10.1007/s00784-018-2337-x.

Khanna, P., & Walt, D. R. (2015). Salivary diagnostics using a portable point-of-service platform: a review. *Clinical therapeutics*, *37*(3), 498–504. https:// doi.org/10.1016/j.clinthera. 2015.02.004.

Wong D. T. (2012). Salivary diagnostics. *Operative dentistry*, *37*(6), 562–570. https://doi.org/10. 2341/12-143-BL.

Chapter 32

Chiarella S. E. (2019). Immunobiologic treatments for severe asthma, atopic dermatitis, and chronic urticaria. *Allergy and asthma proceedings*, *40*(6), 485–489. https://doi.org/10.2500/aap.2019.40.4277.

Mishra, A., Bhalla, S. R., Rawat, S., Bansal, V., Sehgal, R., & Kumar, S. (2007). Standardization and validation of a new atomic absorption spectroscopy technique for determination and quantitation of aluminium adjuvant in immunobiologicals. *Biologicals: journal of the International Association of Biological Standardization*, *35*(4), 277–284. https://doi.org/10.1016/j. biologicals.2007.03.003.

Chapter 33

Levi, Paul A., Rudy, Robert J., Jeong, Y. Natalie, Coleman, Daniel K. (2015-12-29). *Non-Surgical Control of Periodontal Diseases: A Comprehensive Handbook*, Springer. pp. 213–214. ISBN 9783662466230.

Pérez-López, D., Pena-Cristóbal, M., Otero-Rey, E. M., Tomás, I., & Blanco-Carrión, A. (2016). Clinical value of diascopy and other non-invasive techniques on differential diagnosis algorithms of oral pigmentations: A systematic review. *Journal of clinical and experimental dentistry*, *8*(4), e448–e458. https://doi.org/10.4317/jced.53005.

Chapter 34

Tardy, A. L., Pouteau, E., Marquez, D., Yilmaz, C., & Scholey, A. (2020). Vitamins and Minerals for Energy, Fatigue and Cognition: A Narrative Review of the Biochemical and Clinical Evidence. *Nutrients*, *12*(1), 228. https://doi.org/10.3390/nu12010228.

Gutierrez Gossweiler, A., & Martinez-Mier, E. A. (2020). Chapter 6: Vitamins and Oral Health. *Monographs in oral science*, *28*, 59–67. https://doi.org/ 10.1159/000455372.

Abdullah, M., Jamil, R. T., & Attia, F. N. (2021). Vitamin C (Ascorbic Acid). In *StatPearls*. StatPearls Publishing.

Chapter 35

Demmig-Adams, B., López-Pozo, M., Stewart, J. J., & Adams, W. W., 3rd (2020). Zeaxanthin and Lutein: Photoprotectors, Anti-Inflammatories, and Brain Food. *Molecules (Basel, Switzerland)*, *25*(16), 3607. https://doi.org/ 10.3390/molecules25163607.

Mares J. (2016). Lutein and Zeaxanthin Isomers in Eye Health and Disease. *Annual review of nutrition*, *36*, 571–602. https://doi.org/10.1146/annurev-nutr-071715-051110.

Chapter 36

Robert J. Gorlin et al. *Syndromes of the Head and Neck*, 4th edition, Oxford University Press, 2001.

Chapter 37

Seymour R. A. (2013). Antibiotics in dentistry--an update. *Dental update*, *40*(4), 319–322. https://doi.org/10.12968/denu.2013.40.4.319.

Chapter 38

Gupta. B. N, Occupational Diseases of Teeth, *J. soc. Occup. Med.* (1990)40,149-152.

Chapter 39

In *Dental and Maxillofacial radiology*, second edition, Freny R. Karjodkar, Chapter 1, Page:

Chapter 40

A brief history of the periodic table (asbmb.org).
Beta Decay (atomicarchive.com).
Edward J. Hoffman, 62, Professor, Co-Inventor of PET Scan Device - *Los Angeles Times* (latimes.com).
Featured History: Fluoroscopy - UW Radiology (washington.edu).
Gerward, L. Paul Villard and his Discovery of Gamma Rays. *Phys. perspect.* 1, 367–383 (1999). https://doi.org/10.1007/s000160050028.
History of the Gamma Knife - MidMichigan Health.
Paatero, Y. V. and H. Numata. Hallikainen D. History of Panoramic Radiography. *Acta Radiologica*. 1996,37(3P2):441-445. doi:10.1177/02 841851960373P207.
Rutherford's Nuclear World: The Story of the Discovery of the Nucleus | Sections | American Institute of Physics (aip.org).
Synchrotron - Wikipedia.
Website url link: *Structure of atom: Discovery of electrons, protons and neutrons* – Open Teaching Project (padakshep.org).
Who discovered helium? (phys.org).

Chapter 41

Dental and Maxillofacial radiology, second edition, Freny R. Karjodkar.
Oral radiology, Principles and interpretation, Stuart. C. White, Michael. J. Pharoah, *First south asia* edition, In chapter: 1 Physics.

Chapter 42

Dental and Maxillofacial radiology, second edition, Freny R. Karjodkar, Page:60-65.

Chapter 43

Oral radiology, Principles and interpretation, Stuart. C. White, Michael. J. Pharoah, First south asia edition, In chapter: 2 Radiation Biology, Page: 16-28.

Chapter 44

Dental and Maxillofacial radiology, second edition, Freny R. Karjodkar, 2nd edition, 111-128.

Chapter 45

Dental and Maxillofacial radiology, second edition, Freny R. Karjodkar, 2nd edition, 129-144.

Chapter 46

Dental and Maxillofacial radiology, second edition, Freny R. Karjodkar, 2nd edition, 129-144.

Chapter 47

Dental and Maxillofacial radiology, second edition, Freny R. Karjodkar, 2nd edition, 111-128.

Chapter 48

Oral radiology, Principles and interpretation, Stuart. C. White, Michael. J. Pharoah, First south asia edition, In chapter: 7 Intraoral Projections, Page: 91-130.

Chapter 49

Oral radiology, Principles and interpretation, Stuart. C. White, Michael. J. Pharoah, First south Asia edition, In chapter: 7 Intraoral Projections, Page: 91-130.

Chapter 50

Oral radiology, Principles and interpretation, Stuart. C. White, Michael. J. Pharoah, First south Asia edition, In chapter: 10 Panoramic imaging, Page: 166-184.

Chapter 51

Oral radiology, Principles and interpretation, Stuart. C. White, Michael. J. Pharoah, First south Asia edition, In chapter: 4 Digital imaging, Page: 41-62.

Chapter 52

Oral radiology, Principles and interpretation, Stuart. C. White, Michael. J. Pharoah, First south Asia edition, In chapter: 27 Temporomandibular Joint Disorders, Page: 492-523.

Chapter 53

Rogers DC, Tadi P. Intravenous Contrast. [Updated 2021 Apr 25]. In: *StatPearls* [Internet]. Treasure Island (FL): StatPearls Publishing, 2021 Jan-. Available from: https://www.ncbi.nlm.nih.gov/books/NBK557794/.

Chapter 54

Yan, Y., Sun, X., & Shen, B. (2017). Contrast agents in dynamic contrast-enhanced magnetic resonance imaging. *Oncotarget*, *8*(26), 43491–43505. https://doi.org/10.18632/oncotarget.16482.

Chapter 55

Ghorayeb, S. R., Bertoncini, C. A., & Hinders, M. K. (2008). Ultrasonography in dentistry. *IEEE transactions on ultrasonics, ferroelectrics, and frequency control*, *55*(6), 1256–1266. https://doi.org/10.1109/TUFFC.2008.788.

Chapter 56

Xiao, Y. D., Paudel, R., Liu, J., Ma, C., Zhang, Z. S., & Zhou, S. K. (2016). MRI contrast agents: Classification and application (Review). *International journal of molecular medicine*, *38*(5), 1319–1326. https://doi.org/10. 3892/ijmm.2016.2744.

Chapter 57

Dental and Maxillofacial radiology, second edition, Freny R. Karjodkar, 2nd edition, Chapter 14: Computed Tomography, Page: 256-287.

Chapter 58

Dental and Maxillofacial radiology, second edition, Freny R. Karjodkar, 2nd edition, Chapter 14: Magnetic resonance imaging, Chapter 15, Page: 286-323.

Chapter 59

Dental and Maxillofacial radiology, second edition, Freny R. Karjodkar, 2nd edition, Chapter 14: Magnetic resonance imaging, Chapter 15, Page: 286-323.

Chapter 60

Rudi A. J. O Dierckx, *PET and SPECT of Neurobiology systems*, Springer. Page 1-823.

Chapter 61

Rudi A. J. O Dierckx, *PET and SPECT of Neurobiology systems*, Springer. Page 1-823.

Chapter 62

Oral radiology, Principles and interpretation, Stuart. C. White, Michael. J. Pharoah, first south Asia edition, In chapter: 11, Cone beam computed Tomography: volume acquisition Page: 185-198.

Chapter 63

Oral radiology, Principles and interpretation, Stuart. C. White, Michael. J. Pharoah, first south Asia edition, In chapter: 11, Cone beam computed Tomography: volume Preparation Page: 199-213.

Chapter 64

Oral radiology, Principles and interpretation, Stuart. C. White, Michael. J. Pharoah, first south Asia edition, In chapter: 11, Cone beam computed Tomography: volume acquisition Page: 193-198.

Chapter 65

Oral radiology, Principles and interpretation, Stuart. C. White, Michael. J. Pharoah, First south Asia edition, In chapter: 33: Dental implants Page: 630-645.

Chapter 66

Baetke, S. C., Lammers, T., & Kiessling, F. (2015). Applications of nanoparticles for diagnosis and therapy of cancer. *The British journal of radiology*, *88*(1054), 20150207. https://doi.org/10.1259/bjr.20150207.

Dadfar, S. M., Roemhild, K., Drude, N. I., von Stillfried, S., Knüchel, R., Kiessling, F., & Lammers, T. (2019). Iron oxide nanoparticles: Diagnostic, therapeutic and theranostic applications. *Advanced drug delivery reviews*, *138*, 302–325. https://doi.org/10.1016/j.addr.2019.01.005.

Han, X., Xu, K., Taratula, O. & Farsad, K., (2019). Applications of nanoparticles in biomedical imaging. *Nanoscale*, *11*(3), 799–819. https://doi.org/10.1039/ c8nr07769j.

Liu, Y., Bhattarai, P., Dai, Z., & Chen, X., (2019). Photothermal therapy and photoacoustic imaging via nanotheranostics in fighting cancer. *Chemical Society reviews*, *48*(7), 2053–2108. https://doi.org/10.1039/c8cs00618k.

Matea, C. T., Mocan, T., Tabaran, F., Pop, T., Mosteanu, O., Puia, C., Iancu, C., & Mocan, L. (2017). Quantum dots in imaging, drug delivery and sensor applications. *International journal of nanomedicine*, *12*, 5421–5431. https://doi.org/10.2147/IJN.S138624.

Chapter 67

Yi, J., Zhu, J., Zhao, C., Kang, Q., Zhang, X., Suo, K., … Lu, J. (2021). Potential of natural products as radioprotectors and radiosensitizers: opportunities and challenges. *Food & Function*, 12(12), 5204–5218. doi:10.1039/d1fo00525a.

Chapter 68

Oral radiology, Principles and interpretation, Stuart. C. White, Michael. J. Pharoah, First south Asia edition, In chapter: 25, Systemic Diseases Page: 452.

Chapter 69

Schwendicke, F., Samek, W., & Krois, J. (2020). Artificial Intelligence in Dentistry: Chances and Challenges. *Journal of dental research*, *99*(7), 769–774. https://doi.org/10.1177/00220345209 15714.

Machoy, M. E., Szyszka-Sommerfeld, L., Vegh, A., Gedrange, T., & Woźniak, K. (2020). The ways of using machine learning in dentistry. *Advances in clinical and experimental medicine: official organ Wroclaw Medical University*, *29*(3), 375–384. https://doi.org/10.17219/acem/115083.

Chapter 70

Oral radiology, Principles and interpretation, Stuart. C. White, Michael. J. Pharoah, First south Asia edition, In chapter: 15, Quality assurance Page: 250-253.

Chapter 71

Oral radiology, Principles and interpretation, Stuart. C. White, Michael. J. Pharoah, First south Asia edition, In chapter: 25, Infection control Page: 254-258.

Chapter 72

Oral radiology, Principles and interpretation, Stuart. C. White, Michael. J. Pharoah, First south Asia edition, In chapter: 8, Intraoral anatomy, Page: 131-144.

Chapter 73

Oral radiology, Principles and interpretation, Stuart. C. White, Michael. J. Pharoah, First south Asia edition, In chapter: 8, Intraoral anatomy, Page: 144-148.

Chapter 74

Oral radiology, Principles and interpretation, Stuart. C. White, Michael. J. Pharoah, First south Asia edition, In chapter: 17, Principles of radiographic interpretation, Page: 271-284.

Chapter 75

Dental and Maxillofacial radiology, second edition, Freny R. Karjodkar, 2nd edition, chapter 9: Radiographic Films and accessories, Page: 111-128.

Chapter 76

Bhalavat, R., Budrukkar, A., Laskar, S. G., Sharma, D., Mukherji, A., Chandra, M., Mahantshetty, U., Pareek, V., Bauskar, P., & Saraf, S. (2020). Brachytherapy in head and neck malignancies: Indian Brachytherapy Society (IBS) recommendations and guidelines. *Journal of contemporary brachytherapy*, *12*(5), 501–511. https://doi.org/10.5114/jcb.2020.100385.

Kharouta, M., Zender, C., Podder, T., Rezaee, R., Lavertu, P., Fowler, N., Thuener, J., Li, S., Clancy, K., Xu, Z., & Yao, M. (2021). Permanent Interstitial Cesium-131 Brachytherapy in Treating High-Risk Recurrent Head and Neck Cancer: A Prospective Pilot Study. *Frontiers in oncology*, *11*, 639480. https://doi.org/10.3389/fonc.2021.639480.

Murakami, N., Honma, Y., Yoshimoto, S., Shima, S., Kashihara, T., Takahashi, K., Kaneda, T., Inaba, K., Okuma, K., Masui, K., Yoshida, K., Igaki, H., & Itami, J. (2021). Gel spacer to protect carotid artery and reconstructed jejunum in image-guided interstitial brachytherapy for recurrent hypopharyngeal cancer: a technical report. *Journal of contemporary brachytherapy*, *13*(5), 583–587. https://doi.org/10.5114/jcb.2021.109806.

About the Authors

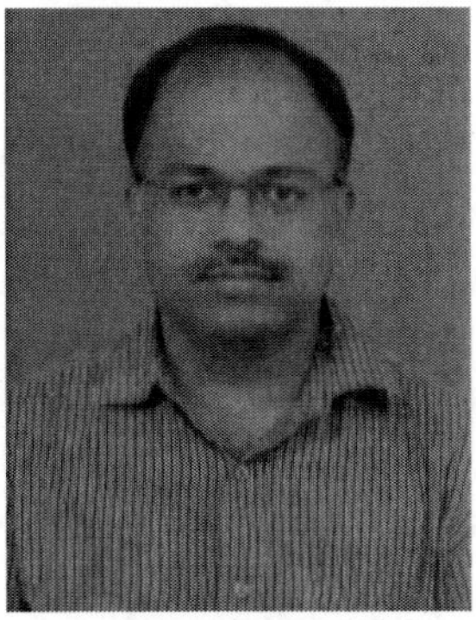

Karthik Rajaram Mohan is currently working as an Associate Professor in the oral medicine and radiology department, Vinayaka Missions Sankarachariyar dental college, Vinayaka Mission's Research Foundation (Deemed to be University), Salem, Tamilnadu, India. He has contributed to various research studies, and case reports in PubMed and Scopus indexed international publications. He has also given national and international scientific presentations. He is currently a member of the associate editorial staff of the Cureus journal of Medical Sciences, a worldwide international Pubmed Central (PMC) indexed journal.

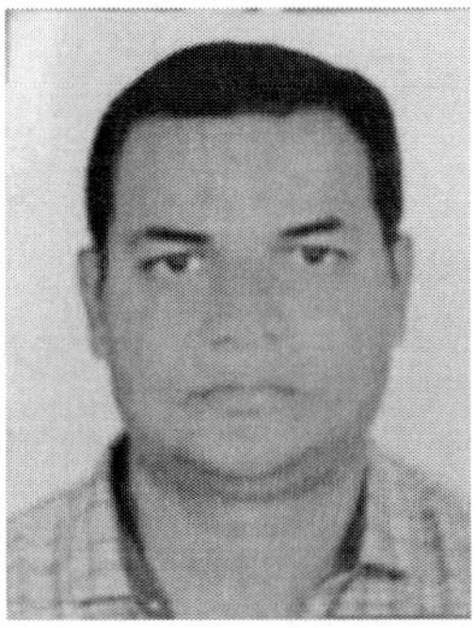

Ravikumar Pethagounder Thangavel - currently working as Head of Department, Department of Oral Medicine and Radiology, Vinayaka Mission's Sankarachariyar dental college, Vinayaka Mission's Research Foundation (Deemed to be University), Salem, Tamilnadu, India. He has presented both national and international scientific papers. In addition, he has contributed to various research studies in Scopus, and Pubmed indexed international Publications.

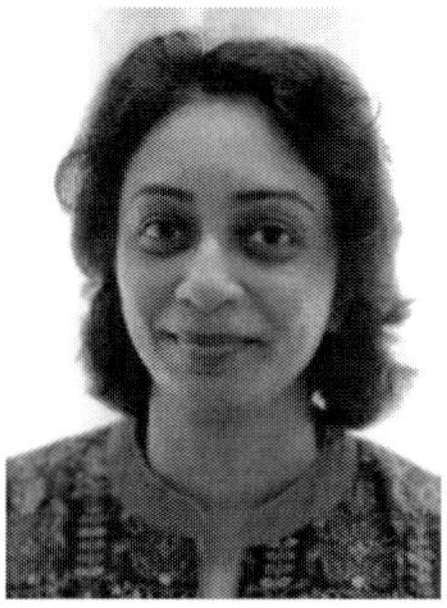

Saramma Mathew Fenn currently working as an associate professor, Department of Oral Medicine and Radiology, Vinayaka Mission's Sankarachariyar dental College, Vinayaka Mission's Research Foundation (Deemed to be University), Salem, Tamilnadu, India. She has completed her PhD in the year 2021. During her postgraduate degree in oral medicine and radiology in 2014, she won the Gold medal. In addition, she has published in a variety of national and international Pubmed and Scopus indexed publications in oral medicine and radiology.

Index